DR. CASS INGRAM

The Miracle of Wild Oregano

KNOWLEDGE
HOUSE
PUBLISHERS

Cover photo by Judy K. Gray, M.S.

Printed in the United States of America

ISBN-10: 1-931078-29-7
ISBN-13: 978-1-931078-29-0

Disclaimer: This book is not intended as a substitute for medical diagnosis or treatment. Anyone who has a serious disease should consult a physician before initiating any change in treatment or before beginning any new treatment.

To order this or additional Knowledge House books call: 1-866-626-5888 or order via the web at: www.knowledgehousepublishers.com

To get an order form send a SASE to:
Knowledge House Publishers
105 East Townline Rd., Unit 116
Vernon Hills, IL 60061

Table of Contents

In the name of the most merciful and gracious God

Introduction

There is a natural medicine that is so powerful that it saves lives. It is a medicine that all people must know about. This is wild oregano. Notice the beautiful plant on the cover of this book. It is like its flower, a white light of this universe. It is a medicine which is specifically mentioned in the divine sources—the actual scriptures and the sayings of the prophets—for human benefit. This natural medicine is more powerful than any drug. It is also more versatile than any man-made substance, including the most highly touted pharmaceutical drugs. What's more, it creates miracles for all to see, if anyone will realize it. Furthermore, far from a modern discovery this is an ancient medicine, in fact, the most ancient known. It is also a key type of medicine mentioned in the Bible as well as by the great prophets, including Moses, Jesus, and Muhammad.

It is no surprise that there are miracles in natural cures. Again, these are the medicines which are created for the benefit of the human being. This is by the almighty creator. This grand Being is seeking to help His human creation. This is through the creation of wild oregano, the most potent cure known. Some people would dispute this. Yet, is there any basis for this dispute?

It is not difficult to believe in miracles, especially in regard to nature. Let us look at some obvious miracles. Consider the skies above and their greatness. No one can understand how the skies are held up and, as well, how they were made. Consider, too, the stars, arranged in profound constellations. That night sky obviously proves the greatness of creation. As well, consider the greatest constellations, the big and little dippers, as if symbols of the mercy of the great creator. The Little Dipper represents the modest blessings of this world, while the Big Dipper represents the endless blessings of the final life. Even so, all people wish to live this life to the fullest. To do so it is necessary to know about natural cures, particularly the wild oregano. There is no way to survive the various trials and tribulations without this powerful substance. It is more critical to survival than all the pharmaceutical drugs combined.

There is proof of the merciful nature of this Being. This is because there truly is a miracle substance for human beings, which will relieve all their agony and despair. There is a profoundly powerful substance, or rather, plant that all people must know about. This is wild oregano.

Those who have used it well know this is a true miracle. This is because it saves lives. These are the lives of people of all backgrounds, races, and status. It saves lives of newborns, infants, toddlers, children, teenagers, adults, and the elderly. It also saves the lives of countless animals, including pet birds, cats, dogs, reptiles, even farm animals. In the United States and Canada alone the lives saved by this invaluable natural substance are countless. Plus, it saves people from endless misery and pain. It causes the return of health when there is no hope. It brings relief when there is no other which can do so. It is just as miraculous as these statements make clear, even more so, despite the fact that skeptics will attempt to deny it.

The only way to determine its power is to use it. Then, a person will quickly become a believer. Yet, why not: why suffer in agony and misery, when there is a substance available to aid the vast needs of humankind and to save this human race from the constant threats of disease and sudden death. Plus this substance is virtually hand-delivered. No human invented or synthesized it. Nor can any human improve upon it. Again, remember the Big Dipper and more, which proves that there is mercy from on High. Yet, will human beings take advantage of it?

For any physician or practitioner who uses wild oregano there is a profound occurrence. Great healings occur. The oregano replaces numerous drugs, including antiseptics, antiinflammatory agents, antibiotics, cough medicines, antacids, and cardiac medicines. Quickly, it is found that this wondrous herb or, rather, spice is far more effective than all such agents. It is determined that it outperforms all known drugs, achieving a vast number of feats. These feats include the fact that it breaks up mucous, halts irritating coughs, culminates allergic reactions, reduces/eliminates pain, reduces swellings, speeds the healing of wounds, obliterates infections, eases angina, helps digestion distress, and strengthens the heart. It clears the sinuses, lungs, and bronchial passages as well as halts diarrhea. No chemical drug has such vast powers, not even remotely so. Rather, this refined substance, this edible oil of wild oregano from the high mountain spice, has more powers than entire categories of drugs. In fact, there are medicines which can't achieve even remotely what the oregano achieves, plus this natural medicine does so, without side effects.

Regardless, how could there be even the concern of side effects? There is no such concern, because this is a wild spice. This means it is a food. Yet, with drugs and vaccines there are vast concerns as well as precautions. Drugs cause countless deaths. Yet, no one has ever died from consuming wild oregano. Even antibiotics, which people often regard as innocuous, cause deaths. Thus, the entire claim or concern of side effects regarding such a substance is ludicrous. Rather, the only side effect is exceptional health, and that is surely an effect all people seek. Regardless, the government lists wild oregano as GRAS, which means "generally regarded as safe." Some people feel they need such a stamp of approval. However, those familiar with wild nature know that with rare exceptions the various whole foods and herbs of nature are entirely safe. Many are even safe for consumption by infants and pregnant women. For instance, in the Middle East pregnant and lactating women routinely consume wild oregano, often daily and even in relatively large quantities, without side effects. Surely, rather than causing any harm wild oregano boosts the health of both the mothers and their babies.

Too, it is one of God's favorite plants. He positions it in highly strategic regions so that it can be of great use to the human race. Its blessed status is obvious, because of how prolific it is in wild nature. It is found primarily in the Mediterranean mountains. It loves high elevations and hates flat or low regions. This is why it is found in the mountains, mainly in remote regions. It requires a highly pure environment. It will not grow naturally in areas of heavy human activity or pollution.

In particular, it thrives in the mountain tops and slopes in the most remote regions on the earth. Here, it thrives on virtually pure rock, where there grows little other vegetation. This is higher than even the most remote mountain villages. In fact, wild oregano thrives best even beyond the trees. It actually grows in the mountains above the tree lines. Here, it thrives virtually up to the mountain peaks. The snow and high elevation doesn't bother it, since it is a tough plant and is also a perennial. This means that its root system can survive the winter to grow again. Thus, this plant loves rocky, barren regions. In contrast, soil, as well as farming, disrupts it.

This plant concentrates energy. This is from the powerful Mediterranean sun. It is also from the rock and the rocky soil. This combination of the sub-tropical sun plus the unique and unaltered soil or rock creates an herbal or, rather, spice powerhouse.

There is great power in this combination. The sun provides light waves, which are highly powerful. These are essentially substances of pure energy without which life would be impossible. The energy from such waves can be trapped within the plant. The rock provides the minerals calcium, phosphorus, and magnesium, which are required for energy production. The rock is whitish gray in color and is never rust or brown colored. The whitish gray color is the result of the dense amounts of calcium and phosphorus. These minerals are vigorously absorbed from the rock by the wild oregano. All this is so that the wild oregano can create certain substances, which have a vast degree of medicinal action.

This is proven by modern research, which shows that wild oregano and, particularly, its extracts—oil of oregano and oregano essence or juice—are among the most powerful curative substances known. The whole crude and freshly ground herb is also highly powerful.

This type of natural medicine has direct and obvious actions on the human body. No other therapeutic agent, natural or synthetic, can match it. Wild oregano is a powerful germicide, antioxidant, fungicide, antihistaminic agent, and antitussive agent. The latter means that it can halt cough. It is also mucolytic, which means that it dissolves mucous deposits.

The germicidal actions are perhaps best known. The wild oregano has been proven to destroy a vast array of germs. This includes bacteria, viruses, fungi, drug-resistant germs, and parasites. It even destroys mites and fleas. Thus, obviously, its powers are vast, far more so than any drug or chemical. Rather, there is even no other herbal medicine, which can match its powers. This may explain why in many countries, such as Turkey, Greece, Lebanon, Syria, Croatia, Bosnia, Serbia, and Palestine, wild oregano is regarded as a "cure-all." For instance, in central Serbia plants of the oregano/thyme family are the only herbs or rather spices which are regarded as "beneficial for all ailments." This is because of the germicidal and antifungal properties of these herbs—and since it is well established that germs are the cause of the majority of diseases this explains the dominating effects of such germ-killing substances.

The plague of fungal infection: power of oregano

The body can easily become overwhelmed by infection. In this regard fungal infections is one of the key infestations. Infection by fungi is a modern epidemic. Actually, globally, billions of humans are afflicted. Moreover, this is not merely surface or localized infections such as athlete's foot, thrush, ringworm, and/or toenail fungus. Rather, this is a plague of systemic infections, where the entire body is infested by these resistant pathogens. What's more, fungal infections are stealth infections, that is there may be few obvious signs of the infestation.

People need to realize the extent of this dilemma. In the modern world virtually no one is immune from fungal infection. Actually, most people never realize the fact that they, too, are likely victims. The fungi create poisons, which intoxicate the system. This may lead to countless symptoms and also much disease. It may be said that fungal infection is the great mimicker, causing countless conditions that are improperly diagnosed.

There are billions of people with fungal overload, and most of them have no obvious symptoms. Typical vague signs and symptoms include indigestion, bloating, chronic constipation, chronic diarrhea, intestinal cramps, foggy feeling, tiredness, vaginal itch, vaginal discharge, urethral pain, bladder disorders, sensitivity to chemicals/odors, depression, impotence, and low libido. More obvious signs include white, yellowish, or gray coating on the tongue, leukoplakia, alopecia, dandruff, seborrhea, vitiligo, athlete's foot, ringworm, jock itch, and toenail/fingernail fungus. Mediterranean-source oil of wild oregano obliterates fungi (plural for fungus). The oil has a high penetrating power for attacking and destroying fungi, including deep infestations, where these germs deeply invade the membranes as well as skin.

Yet, even so, some infections require additional therapy. Often, for ideal results a combination of spice oils may be necessary. This is in addition to the oil of wild oregano. This is in stubborn cases, where the fungus is resistant, where it deeply and persistently invades the body. This combination of fungal cleansing oils may include oil of wild oregano, oil of wild bay leaf, oil of wild sage, cinnamon oil, and cumin oil. Thus, in stubborn cases for ideal results the therapy must include oil of wild oregano and a complex of the aforementioned oils. Ideally, this can be taken as oils under the tongue. Or, these may be taken as capsules, which contain the dessicated spice oils. For best results these oils/capsules must be taken two or more times daily. In tough cases it may be necessary to take these doses four or five times daily. Also, in such high doses there is need to support the intestines with healthy bacterial supplements.

Spice oils, such as oil of wild oregano, are potent antifungal agents. Clinically, these oils truly help purge fungi from the intestines, blood, genitals, and internal organs. Not all spice oils exert this effect. Nor do all herbal oils. Only certain of these oils are truly effective. The most effective of all is the oil of wild oregano, followed by in order of potency oil of cumin, oil of bay leaf, oil of cinnamon, and oil of sage. Yet another moderately powerful antifungal oil is oil of wild myrtle. This offers the unique benefit of being mild enough to use topically in sensitive areas such as the inner thighs near the genitals, on the genitals themselves, and about the eyes. Thyme oil is also highly antifungal, but it is caustic. Even so, the most supreme of all antifungal agents is oil of wild oregano from the true wild Mediterranean spice. This is safe for human consumption.

In contrast to these highly effective antifungal oils there are other aromatic oils such as oils of cayenne, basil, coriander, rosemary, mint, and lavender. All these are relatively weak antifungal agents. Thus, it is important to know which oils are truly antifungal agents and to use only such oils for this therapy.

The greatest antibacterial agent known

Wild oregano is highly destructive against bacteria. Testing shows that all bacteria succumb to it. There is no synthetic substance that can match it. This natural oil is the most broad-spectrum 'antibiotic' known. Even so, it is well known that certain powerful forces dislike such statements. Yet, this doesn't mean it isn't true. According to studies at Georgetown University and Celsus Labs Mediterranean-source wild oregano oil, that is the original and researched brand—the brand which has undergone extensive research at Georgetown University, Washington, D. C.—is so potent that it even neutralizes virtually all known germs. More importantly, it kills common pathogens—such as E. coli, strep, salmonella, the cold virus, the flu virus, and staph—which cause human disease. This is determined by the governments' own research published by the FDA in the *Journal of Food Protection*, 1999. Here, it was discovered that wild oregano obliterates tough germs which cause food poisoning, including staph, salmonella, and E. coli 0157:H7, the latter being a mutant. Moreover, it does so without side effects.

The lifesaving powers of this natural substance are demonstrated by the fact that it can do what drugs are incapable of achieving. This is the destruction of drug resistant germs. The oil emulsified in extra virgin olive oil was recently tested against drug resistant staph, in fact, MRSA. It is MRSA, which is methicillin-resistant *Staphyloccocus aureus*, which is the plague of modern medicine. In the United States and Canada alone some 50,000 people die every year from this infection. All these deaths are preventable.

MRSA is the type of staph which causes much disability and death in hospitalized patients. Incredibly, while there is no drug which can reliably kill it this germ is readily destroyed by spice oils. This is through the internal and topical use of the oil as well as the use of the multiple spice spray containing oil of wild oregano and other phenol-rich spice oils.

Since in particular the oil of wild oregano in a high or super strength form can obliterate this essentially 'incurable' infection, then, obviously killing other bacteria is a minor issue. This is confirmed by scientific studies published in a wide range of journals, including the *Journal of Agricultural and Food Chemistry* and *Molecular and Cellular Biochemistry,* have demonstrated that, in fact, oil of wild oregano obliterates all bacteria against which it is tested.

Again, all the bacteria succumb to it. No drug even has this power. Only the power of nature can achieve this incredible result. People should take note of this fact: there are no synthetic substances which match it. For instance, in a test done at Georgetown University and published by H. Preuss the oil of wild oregano was demonstrated to kill five hardy bacteria which cause human disease, including staph, klebsiella, mycobacterium, E. coli, and anthrax. In contrast, again, no antibiotic demonstrates such power. In a study performed by Italian investigators 13 different bacteria were destroyed by the oil. Again, at Georgetown University drug resistant staph were destroyed, in this instance, in mice. The study, published in *Molecular and Cellular Biochemistry*, proved that wild oregano oil worked equally as well as a powerful drug, Vancomycin, in preventing the deaths of mice from the infection. Rather, according to the investigators the wild oregano oil was superior to the drug, since it proved less toxic, the drug causing a kind of immune suppression in the mice.

Studies at Celsus Labs demonstrate another unique action of spice oils. This is in a base of truly natural substances which form a kind of thin white liquid or emulsion. This emulsion is a spray that is thoroughly absorbed into the tissues. It is also readily disseminated into the air. This is in regard to killing airborne, as well as surface, bacteria. This emulsified spray is highly effective in killing airborne germs, including bacteria, viruses, and molds. Also, when the emulsion is mixed with hand soap, too, this results in the killing of harmful germs. The emulsion contains a combination of spice oils.

Oregano oil cream in a honey/propolis base is also a powerful natural medicine. Evaluations on humans have demonstrated that a 6% essential oil-based cream with wild oils of oregano, St. John's wort, and lavender is effective against skin infections such as acne and impetigo. This is a soothing way to apply the wild oregano to skin lesions and irritations. Also, the cream has significant powers in preventing skin aging. Here, it helps boost the skin's internal healing mechanisms and therefore helps prevent and reverse age-related damage. In addition, it is an ideal emollient to use on sun damaged skin, including acute sunburns. Thus, clearly, wild oregano and spice oil-based natural medicines are a boon for the human race.

Even so, some people don't believe in these medicines. Often, these are people who believe mainly in chemicals. They may well be heavy smokers and drinkers as well as people who take multiple medications. So, rather than the real effectiveness or science behind natural medicine it is belief systems that have much to do with peoples' attitudes. That natural medicine is effective is beyond question. Drug companies attempt to dispute otherwise. Yet, are the medicines made by these companies themselves effective? Are they useful in the actual treatment and reversal of disease? In fact, with rare exceptions there are no such medicines.

The federal government seems to agree with these conclusions. At several institutions it has studied or investigated wild oregano. The involved institutions include the USDA, Pentagon, and FDA. Government studies include the use of oregano oil to kill food-borne pathogens as well as the addition of the oil and spice as food preservatives. At the USDA a wild oregano-based food film has been patented. The oil from the original research by the FDA was precisely the type which is now being scrutinized by these same federal people. Plus, all the interest and research regarding the powers of this spice oil has been achieved by the scrutinized company. Despite this, as this book goes to press the federal government is funding new research regarding oregano at Delaware State University.

Other governments are taking note of oregano's powers. In Algeria a team of researchers found that wild oregano oil is more powerful than pesticides in preventing infestation of cereals by grain beetles. Also, as mentioned previously the USDA has determined that oregano oil and other spice oils, impregnated into biofilms, help prevent food poisoning in processed foods. Furthermore, the Canadian government is investigating this spice oil's powers. In 2005 this government published a study comparing the destructive actions of both radiation and oregano oil against bacteria. The study demonstrated that oregano oil had a direct destructive effect against E. coli, a major cause of food spoilage as well as human disease. This research, published in the *Journal of Food Protection*, demonstrated that the oregano oil was the superior of the two treatments, causing systematic destruction of the bacterial cell walls. Moreover, this was the highly toxic strain, known as E. coli 0157:H7, which, again, the oregano oil destroyed.

Considerable money is being spent by the U. S. federal government on spice oil research. This research is funded strictly by tax-payers. For instance, some $10,000 was given by the government to the Maine Organic Farmer and Gardener's Association in Unity, Maine, to study the effect of feeding oregano to sheep to prevent parasitic infections. More dominantly, the federal government set aside some $450,000 to test the powers of wild oregano and other spices against common food borne pathogens, with the initial findings being published in the *Journal of Food Protection*. According to government researchers, the original purpose of the study was to "prove" that the use of oregano or any other spice as a natural medicine is "a useless endeavor." This is stated categorically by the lead researcher of the study, Dr. Frances Ann Draughon. Despite this, the government has made clear, oregano truly works in the prevention of food poisoning. Thus, any antagonism by the government against wild oregano therapy is purely hypocritical.

Chapter One

The Strength of Nature

Some people think that drugs are powerful. Even so, there are no synthetic substances which are as powerful as natural medicines. Regardless, drugs were originally derived from natural substances. So, which is more powerful, the original source or a laboratory fabrication?

The ancients knew better. In early eras there was no pharmaceutical cartel to "control" the information. Regarding wild oregano consider the ancient Greeks. They called this plant or the "delight" or "pleasure" of the mountains *oro ganos*. Thus, they realized its essential nature for human health. This authority maintained by wild oregano is proven by the discovery of an ancient Grecian shipwreck off the coast of Chios in the Aegean Sea. Incredibly, the cargo of the shipwreck was mainly olive oil flavored with wild oregano.

Again, this was the entire cargo. It consisted of amphora containing an oregano-infused olive oil, which was distinct to the people of Chios. There were some 350 such amphora found on the wreck. The shipwreck was about 2400 years old. This was precious cargo, which proves that for this ancient society, which boasts the still-admired Hippocrates or "father of medicine," food is truly the best medicine.

The most prominent studies available prove that food is curative. In contrast, when animals were fed synthetic food they either became deathly ill or died, while any group of such animals fed the natural alternatives thrive.

Drugs are a major cause of degenerative disease. More importantly, in the Western world they are the key cause of sudden death. Then, are any natural, wholesome foods the primary cause of such disease and death? Furthermore, is there any natural food-based herb or spice, such as garlic, onion, basil, oregano, thyme, sage, rosemary, fenugreek, coriander, mustard, cumin, cinnamon, and clove, which is a major cause of degeneration, let alone death? There are no such whole food substances, which cause such devastation.

It is on the contrary, since these substances, in fact, save lives. They also prevent great diseases. Here, the powers of wild oregano in this regard are made clear. There can be no doubt about it, in particular, that this food or spice is a lifesaving substance and functions in a manner opposite of drugs. Its greatest powers in this regard relate to its antiseptic properties, that is its germ-killing powers, which are considerable. This is why it has such a positive influence on the whole body. Germs are a major cause of human disease. They are opportunists and thus attack the body when it is weak. What's more, oregano strengthens immunity while also killing germs. In contrast, synthetic drugs depress immunity, while creating mutant germs, which further disable the immune system.

Anyone who is worried about the potential harm of this natural spice oil is wasting his or her time. The great harm to humanity is from synthetic chemicals, not natural spice oils. Rather, it is the spice oils which are the real source of aid, the great purging agents—the great cures—used by the ancients.

Yet, too, these are cures which are also mentioned in the original scriptures.

That oregano oil is lifesaving has been known for centuries. In this modern era research began regarding its powers early in the 20th century. In 1910 it was W. H. Martindale who determined the ultimate power of wild oregano. After extensive research he stated categorically that "the essential oil of oregano is the most powerful plant-derived antiseptic known." It was Martindale who first showed that oregano oil is 26 times more potent than synthetic phenol, then known as carbolic acid. Thus, clearly, there is no drug nor even categories of drugs which can match such power. In fact, the relatively weak carbolic acid was the drug or synthetic version of carvacrol and thymol, the main active ingredients of oregano oil.

In 1918 Cavel, working at the Pasteur institute, studied a number of essential oils regarding their ability to sterilize septic water. Here, he inoculated water from septic tanks with beef broth, dramatically increasing microbial growth. He then added various essential oils. Oregano oil, he determined, was so powerful that in a one-tenth of a percent concentration, that is one in 1000, it sterilized septic water. In 1977 Belaniche, while investigating a number of natural compounds, gave oregano oil the highest marks. Said the researcher regarding its germ killing powers in comparison to all antiseptic oils "oregano is the best of the best." Furthermore, regarding oregano oil and similar spice oils according to the world renown Jean Valnet, M.D., these "proved to be many times more effective at killing pathogenic microorganisms than antibiotics." Valnet, a French physician, routinely prescribed spice oils and found them effective in a wide range of conditions, including lung disease, cardiovascular disease, arthritis, kidney disease and intestinal disorders. The work of these early researchers is confirmed by the latest research, which will be described throughout this book.

The most powerful antiviral agent

Wild oregano destroys viruses. This is particularly true of the steam distilled oil. This oil does so both on and in the body. Viruses known to be killed by oil of wild oregano include herpes viruses, hepatitis viruses, the cold virus, the flu virus, Newcastle virus, and respiratory syncytial virus. According to English investigators the oil is even capable of inhibiting the growth of HIV/AIDS viruses.

Studies prove that the antiviral powers of wild oil of oregano are exceptional. In a study using the original wild Mediterranean brand in an extra virgin olive oil base and performed by Microbiotest, oil of wild oregano was found to essentially decimate both the cold and flu viruses. This was an in vitro study, meaning it was done inside cells. In this instance the viruses were used to infect chicken embryo cells, the latter being incubated to speed viral growth.

First, the corona virus, a common cause of colds, was evaluated. Per milliliter of material some 5.5 million viruses were detected, as published in *Antiviral Research*. After treatment with a small amount, that is .01%, of the oil only a mere 4,000 or so viruses were detected. This is a 99.9% kill. What's more, this occurred in a mere 20 minutes. A combination of oils of wild oregano and sage, along with cumin and cinnamon oil, dessicated into a powder, achieved an even more dramatic effect. Here, in 20 minutes a 100% kill was achieved. This dessicated spice extract is available in capsule form as a combination of the dried essence of wild oregano and sage plus cumin and cinnamon.

The same was achieved with the flu virus, although this virus proved tougher. It took a 1% solution to achieve in 20 minutes a 99.7% kill by the oil of wild oregano, and an even more vigorous kill was achieved by the multiple spice combination. A variant of bird flu was also tested. The bird flu viruses are extremely powerful as well as resistant. Here, for a 99.7% kill a 25% solution of the oil of wild oregano was required. This is not to claim that the oil is a cure for all such diseases. Rather, it is simply to state that these are the exact results from scientific studies.

People can determine for themselves the implications. Moreover, the government has no right to condemn these results as insufficient. Can the government provide proof of any other substance which offers even remotely similar powers? Furthermore, the complete destruction of septic water has obvious implications, as does the comparison of French physicians, such as Valnet, of oregano oil versus antibiotics, that is the statement that the oregano oil is vastly superior to such drugs. Such a statement makes infinite sense, since, while antibiotics kill only specific germs, natural antiseptics, such as extracts of oil of wild oregano, bay leaf, and sage, as well as cumin and cinnamon, obliterate entire categories of germs, in fact, multiple categories.

The most effective antifungal agent

There will be much said throughout this book about fungi. It is against fungal disorders, where the wild oregano is exceptional. This is related to the nature of fungal infections. These infections are chronic. They are also deep-seated. In other words, they are well entrenched in the body. Fungi can penetrate virtually any tissue. Here, they cause tissue invasion and thus great inflammation. This ultimately leads to disease. There is need for a substance, which can be consumed regularly and in relatively large quantities. This is why the wild oregano is so invaluable.

Again, fungi are a major cause of chronic disease. So, there is a vast need for a substance capable of safely eradicating disease-causing fungi from the body. Wild oregano oil, as well as other heat-producing spice oils, are such substances. Preliminary studies demonstrate that such oils obliterate fungi, even from the internal organs. This is based largely on studies in test tubes and petri dishes, yet, animal studies have confirmed this. So have a multitude of human cases.

It is not easy to eradicate fungi from the body. Yet, wild oregano has this power. It destroys the fungi directly, plus it prevents these organisms from becoming reestablished.

In modern medicine the medications are minimal which are effective against fungi. Plus, the majority of these medications are highly toxic, causing potential liver and kidney damage. Other such drugs are effective temporarily, that is they do kill the fungus; however, the fungus ultimately returns and the infection is reestablished. This is why the oregano oil, along with the dessicated multiple spice extract, is so valuable. It tends to destroy the fungus permanently. This is as a result of taking the oil consistently for a sufficient period. What's more, unlike pharmaceutical agents it can be taken for a prolonged period, without concern of toxicity. Furthermore, it can be taken on a daily basis, that is until the fungal infestation is eradicated. Furthermore, after this it can be taken on a daily or weekly basis to prevent fungal recurrence. Plus, it has the versatility of being both a topical and internal agent.

Fungi have the capacity for deep tissue invasion. The purpose is to maintain a permanent presence in the tissues. These fungi are not easy to dislodge. To ultimately destroy the fungi requires patience, along with the use of natural antifungal treatments, which can be taken over a prolonged period.

Even so, the treatment for fungal disorders should be broad spectrum. It should not just be wild oregano products. Diet plays a crucial role, as does exercise and fresh air. If the surroundings are contaminated with fungi, then, the person will readily become reinfected. This is particularly true for those with compromised immune systems. If there is no sunshine, then, the tissues are weakened and fungi will thrive. If there is an excess of sugar in the diet, this will feed fungi. All this must be taken into consideration in achieving a true cleanse, that is cure, of fungal infestation.

Whole pure food is important in eliminating fungi. There are certain foods, in fact, which do the opposite, that is they increase fungal growth. While toxic foods will be covered in detail later in this book the primary foods which feed fungi are refined sugar, white flour, white rice, and highly sweet fruit products. Regarding fruit or fruit products the ones that most greatly feed fungi are apples, pears, apple juice, pear juice, and orange juice. Sour oranges are preferable over sweet oranges. Yet, in particular it is the heavily refined sources of sugar, such as the clarified juices, which accelerate fungal growth.

Bowel cleansing is important in the elimination of fungi. This is because the bowels are the main site of fungal infestation. In fact, the entire intestinal tract may become infested. Various wild herbal extracts, wild greens, and wild berries can be used in the cleansing process. In particular, wild herbal extracts, as well as extracts of spices, are powerful stimulants for the liver and gallbladder. It is these organs which are responsible for bile synthesis and storage, moreover, it is the bile which is the body's natural intestinal cleansing agent. As well, wild raw greens extracts are highly potent for stimulating bile production.

Bile itself is a natural antifungal agent. Great quantities of bile are needed to keep the intestines clean, and, of course, it is the intestines, where the fungi largely hold residence. To produce these great quantities of bile specific foods and extracts must be taken. Normal food will never achieve this. Foods and extracts which cause the massive production of bile are relatively few. Such foods/extracts include black seed oil, extra virgin olive oil, pure fresh-squeezed lemon juice (when combined with either of the aforementioned oils), raw apple cider vinegar (again when combined with such oils), wild raw greens extracts, turmeric extract, silymarin extract, juice of wild thistle, oil of cilantro, oil of fennel, oil of cumin, dark-colored berries, and dark-colored berry extracts. Actual supplements to take which achieve this bile movement and therefore consistent intestinal cleansing include oil of cumin in extra virgin olive oil, oil of cilantro in extra virgin olive oil, liver-cleansing capsules containing cilantro (or coriander), turmeric, cumin, wild raw greens drops, wild raw dark-colored berries drops, crude cold-pressed extra virgin olive oil, and cold-pressed black seed oil.

Again, for best results in the destruction of fungi the wild oregano therapy should be combined with natural cleansing. The liver and gallbladder must be continuously stimulated, while the colon must be consistently flushed. Again, this is through the stimulation of bile synthesis, which is essential in the ultimate cleansing of all fungi from the body. Note: most of the aforementioned bile stimulants are found in the total body purging agent, which is available as a 12-ounce bottle and which contains the wild greens plus spice oils, extra virgin olive oil, and black seed oil. Also, there is a triple wild raw greens concentrate as drops under the tongue and an eight wild berries concentrate as maximum strength wild berries. There are also liver cleansing capsules containing cumin, coriander (that is cilantro), and turmeric. All these supplements are the ideal ones to take, along with the oil of wild oregano and similar wild oregano supplements.

Some people might feel confused about this, that is regarding which supplements to buy. Know that this is not about brand names but rather it is about guiding people to the quality they need, so they can efficiently get well and also stay well. To do this hold firmly to the guidance in this book. The purging agent must be a combination of the aforementioned. The wild greens must be raw, being used as drops under the tongue. The berries must also be raw as well as wild and should contain wild raw blackberry, black raspberry, chokecherry, and similar extracts. These rich-colored berries elicit bile production but only do so in the raw state. There may also be raw wild greens of various types, such as fireweed, nettles, and dandelion, as 12-ounce bottles in a base of essence of wild oregano.

Beets also stimulate bile flow. There are raw beet tablets on the market, but they are difficult to find. If these are unavailable, cooked beets are an option, as is beet juice, ideally from organic sources.

There is also the issue of the healthy bacteria. For the health of the gut and the liver, as well as the immune system, these bacteria are essential. In addition, these bacteria help combat the overgrowth of fungi, especially yeast. Thus, the antifungal protocol should include the intake of such bacteria, either through high quality fermented milk products or healthy bacterial supplements—or both. The Ecologic 500 Strain is an example of a high quality healthy bacterial supplement, although there are a number of excellent products on the market. The Ecologic 500 Strain is particularly desirable, because of its high rate of implantation in the gut plus the quality of its sources which are non-animal. This strain of bacteria is derived from plants. It is also extensively researched and proven to have a high degree of implantation.

All such therapies are effective in the elimination of the fungi. Yet, it must always be remembered that these germs are tough and that they create chronic infections. Thus, it may take a considerable amount of effort and time to fully purge them. For the eradication of chronic fungal infection patience is the rule. It may take weeks or months to fully purge it.

Anti-allergy powers

Wild oregano is a lifesaver against allergic reactions. It halts such reactions as well as prevents them. This is because this spice is a potent antihistaminic agent. When taken vigorously, it can essentially halt and reverse allergic shock, that is the shock reaction, which results from eating a toxic or allergenic food. This includes reactions such as peanut allergy and reactions to drugs such as penicillin. Even the dire reaction to bee stings can be halted by this oil. No such reactions need be fatal, that is as long as the wild high grade oil of oregano (blue label brand) is available.

One ideal way to take the wild oregano for halting allergic reactions is through drops under the tongue. As soon as an allergic reaction develops the drops should be taken and as often as necessary. Usually, a few drops under the tongue taken once or twice stops the reaction, but, again, this may be done as often as needed until all reactions are halted. Another option is to take the crushed whole herb in a capsule or the oil as a gelatin capsule. Too, the oil and the crushed herb may be taken preventively, for instance, in the case of children with peanut allergy or other people who are at a high risk for sudden allergic reactions.

The crude herb is also an anti-allergy supplement. The antihistaminic powers may largely be a result of oregano's rich supply of flavonoids, notably quercitin. Regarding the latter it is well known that this flavonoid is a histamine blocker. This blockade is invaluable for reversing both allergic intolerance to food and also allergies to inhalants. The crude herb plus the oil of oregano are an invincible pair for halting and preventing allergic reactions. This includes life-threatening reactions to foods such as peanuts and shrimp. Also, those who are allergic to drugs, as well as bee stings, would greatly benefit from the regular intake of both these forms of wild oregano.

Regarding the oil it is the phenolic compounds, which account for its dependable powers. Like flavonoids, phenols are also powerful antihistamines. Plus, these chemicals are antiseptics, notably, they are powerful antifungal agents. This largely explains their effectiveness as antihistaminic agents or more particularly as agents for reversing sinus and bronchial disorders. This is because such disorders are usually caused by mold/fungal infection. These infections cause inflammation and therefore the release of histamine. Obviously, when such infections are purged, then, histamine release is culminated. This killing of the molds and fungi is an efficient way to halt allergy symptoms. Thus, there are two mechanisms of actions operating simultaneously: the blockage of histamine release and the killing of the causative invaders.

As mentioned previously there is a third mechanism of action, which is the flavonoids, which are themselves antihistaminic. These flavonoids are only found in the whole crude herb—as found in vegetable gelatin capsules, along with *Rhus coriaria*—as well as the supercritical/carbon dioxide extract (emulsified in extra virgin olive oil).

Wild oregano versus parasites

This natural spice is moderately effective against parasites. In particular, it is highly destructive against giardia and amebas. It is also effective against *Blastocystis hominis*. The crude herb, along with *Rhus coriaria*, has action against tapeworms.

Parasites are all about us. They are found in vast numbers in the soil and water. They are also found on food, particularly vegetables. In uncooked meat they abound, and some of these parasites can even survive the cooking process. Parasites are major contaminants of pork and bear meat. People who eat these meats are usually thoroughly contaminated. This is largely because, even after such meats are cooked, the parasites remain viable. In addition, those who travel overseas frequently and freely consume the food, especially travelers to Mexico, Turkey, China, Korea, and India, are likely to suffer from extreme parasitic infestation. There is no way to have ideal health until these parasites are purged. They cause a great deal of toxicity in the human body. These parasites cause vast inflammation to such a degree that they initiate actual diseases: heart disease, high blood pressure, arthritis, psoriasis, eczema, lupus, and cancer. Furthermore, parasites drain energy from the body and, therefore, are a major cause of chronic fatigue syndrome. They may also attack the brain and cause neurological conditions such as multiple sclerosis, Parkinson's disease, ALS (Lou Gehrig's disease), and Alzheimer's disease. They are also the major factor in diseases of the digestive tract such as Crohn's disease, ulcerative colitis, spastic bowel, liver abscess, pancreatitis, chronic constipation, and diverticulitis.

When these parasites are destroyed, the body is greatly liberated. To destroy them all forms of wild oregano must be used, that is the whole crude herb with *Rhus coriaria*, the oil, and the watery essence or juice. Also, a purging agent should be taken that contains oils of fennel and coriander plus black seed oil and wild greens. In order to destroy the parasites the purging agent and the oregano supplements must be taken for about one to two months. This system of purging may be taken along with a regular diet or a juice fast. If doing a juice fast, do this only for a maximum of two weeks. Ideally, during this fast also eat raw pumpkinseeds, which greatly aid in the expelling of parasites, especially worms. The raw pumpkinseeds can be mixed in raw honey or eaten naturally. The amount needed to facilitate the purge is about a pound or two daily. The raw pumpkinseed should be eaten for about five days. Then, pure raw juices alone can be resumed.

The mite killer

Yes, it is true. Mites cause human diseases. It is well known that people can be allergic to these insects and this, then, leads to allergic sensitivity. It is also well known that asthma can be caused, or rather, aggravated by mites. However, what is less known is that mites can cause specific diseases by actually infecting human tissue. Here, these insects mainly infect the surface tissues, that is the hair, scalp, and skin. They burrow into these tissues causing inflammation and ultimately disease. Disorders and diseases caused by mite infestation include male pattern baldness, alopecia, dandruff, seborrhea, psoriasis, acne, and rosacea. Also, of course, scabies is caused exclusively by mites, this organism being once famously known as the *itch mite*.

How to use wild oregano

Wild oregano is highly diverse. It can be used in dozens of ways, in and on the body. The wild oregano is effective both as the whole crude herb and various extracts. Each type of wild oregano has specific functions, as will be demonstrated as follows:

Steam distilled oil

This is the most popular form of wild oregano extract. This is made strictly through steam. The steam is permeated through wild oregano leaves to produce a slowly extracted oil. As mentioned previously for killing germs this is the most powerful form. The steam extract is high in powerful germicides known as phenols as well as terpenes.

The essential oil is too caustic to take internally. Thus, this oil must be emulsified in extra virgin olive oil to ensure both safety and effectiveness. Such a supplement is safe to take on a daily basis. Even so, for prevention it is sufficiently powerful that it may even be taken occasionally, like twice weekly.

This is the premier type of wild oregano extract. Studies show that this type is the most powerful one for killing germs. For instance, a number of studies show that, through steam distillation, the germ killing powers are enhanced, while cold pressed versions, such as oils extracted by supercritical processes, are much weaker as germ killers.

The steam distilled type is also the ideal form for sublingual administration. This is the means to distribute the wild oregano oil directly into the bloodstream. Through this germs can be rapidly destroyed, since the blood will carry the oil of wild oregano throughout the body. For infections of the gut the sublingual use is even more effective than merely swallowing the oil. This is because the blood supply that feeds the gut arises from outside this organ. By taking the oil sublingually the medicinal substances are then absorbed into the blood to be transported to the gut via its blood supply. This is known as the mesenteric arterial system. With the oregano in this blood system it may be delivered to the gut wall, where it exerts its potent action. The blue label material is made exclusively through steam distillation and thus offers the most powerful action against both germs and inflammation.

Aromatic water (juice)

This is another steam extract of wild oregano. The steam interacts with certain compounds in the wild oregano leaves and extracts them. These compounds are high in oxygen. Thus, the juice is the most oxygenated form of wild oregano available. This oxygen is bound to the wild spice molecules and is, therefore, readily used by the body.

In particular, this oxygen is much needed by the brain. What's more, this essence is well absorbed into neurological tissue, much more so than the oil. Thus, this is the ideal form for the reversal of neurological disorders, including Alzheimer's disease, Parkinson's disease, Lou Gehrig's disease, multiple sclerosis, dementia, myasthenia gravis, paralysis, epilepsy, autism, and brain cancer.

The aromatic essence is a top source of natural oxygen. Thus, for anyone with low level disorders of the brain and nervous system, such as mental fog, confusion, sluggish mental activity, and attention deficit, this form of wild oregano is ideal. It is also a potent agent for increasing physical strength. Thus, it is of great value for people who are athletic.

People who are low in oxygen have a curious sign on their bodies, which is related to the moons on the fingernails. These moons are found usually on all fingers as well as the thumb. For virtually all people, however, the pinky or fifth finger is usually lacking in this. So, this finger can be ignored. However, a lack of moons on the first, second, and third fingers of the body is a sign of low oxygen utilization in the cells. In such an instance there may be a sluggish thyroid function (see *Eat Right for Your Metabolic Type*, same author, Knowledgehousepublishers.com). Here, the oregano juice must be taken, along with the oil of wild oregano and the wild raw triple greens flushing agent, since wild raw greens, like oregano juice, are rich in natural oxygen. What's more, these wild raw greens are a top source of riboflavin, which is needed for oxygen utilization within cells. The oregano juice is particularly ideal for oxygenation, since the oxygen-rich compounds in it readily cross the blood-brain barrier. In addition, vitamin E helps increase oxygen use, and a lack of moons may indicate the deficiency of this vitamin. Yet, regarding supplementation, the use of commercial vitamin E is inappropriate. This is because it is derived from genetically engineered materials and therefore is potentially toxic. A superior choice is vitamin E extracted from sunflower seeds. This, of course, is non-genetically engineered. Thus, this is a safe way to increase the oxygen-carrying capacity of the body.

Crude crushed herb, combined with Rhus coriaria (village formula)

This is the original crude wild oregano formula, made by the mountain villagers some 4000 years ago. Somehow, these villagers found that the addition of these two wild foods, that is the leaves of wild oregano plus the berries of wild rhus, made a perfect food additive. This is available today as capsules and also a bulk powder. It is a whole raw food, which is highly versatile. It can be used in cooking as well as taken orally as a supplement. This is the best type to give regularly to children as well as pets. Look for the type containing a combination of wild crushed oregano, wild *Rhus coriaria* plus organic onion and garlic. This original village formula is highly tasty and thus is an ideal addition to food.

Carbon dioxide extract (flavonoid-rich)

This is the truly cold-extracted form of wild oregano. Thus, this is a raw kind of oregano extract. This means the wild-source oregano enzymes are intact.

The means of extraction is the use of carbon dioxide under high pressure. This leads to the extraction of the various natural chemicals in the oregano, including the flavonoids, phenols, and polyphenols. The enzymes are also extracted. Thus, this carbon dioxide extract is a whole raw food.

The flavonoids offer a powerful antiinflammatory action. Plus, they are anti-allergy. They are also antitumor. Thus, the carbon dioxide extract is the ideal type for severe inflammatory disorders and cancer as well as certain diseases related to allergy such as asthma.

Flavonoids are also antiviral. The flavonoids in oregano exert potent antiviral activity, both internally and externally. The carbon dioxide extract is a powerful topical antiviral agent for use against, for instance, warts. Usually, the application of this oil will cause the destruction of warts rapidly, within a week or less.

Emulsified (mycelized) oil of oregano

The emulsified oil is a type of oregano oil which is made soluble in water. This is known as mycelization. A mycel is a chemical bond between oil and water so that the two mix. This causes the end product to dissolve well in water. Mycelized oil of oregano is the ideal type for children and pets. It mixes well in any juice; it also mixes perfectly in milk.

Oregano oil's main site of action is the watery part of the body, meaning the blood and cellular fluids. So, a water soluble type is ideal, that is for delivering the power of the oregano oil, where it is needed.

In England doctors/practitioners are particularly fond of this water soluble type. They use it in the treatment of candida infections. One practitioner reported that the mycelized form of oregano in particular greatly increased symptoms of "die off." This is a positive result. It means that the oregano oil is causing the killing of noxious germs. Again, this is because the water soluble type of oregano is able to penetrate into the deepest regions of the body, including the greatest depths of the internal organs. Through this deep penetration vile germs are routed out of the body. Thus, for difficult cases of fungal infection or for any type of chronic infection it may be necessary to supplement the regular type of oil of oregano with the water soluble type.

Vacuum-dried oil of wild oregano bound to maltodextrin: the "dessicated" multiple spice complex

This is, perhaps, the most powerful type of wild oregano known. Tests prove that this vacuum-dried oil is even more powerful than the steam distilled type in thoroughly killing germs. In one study against the cold virus it was found that this extract killed, in merely 20 minutes, 100% of all cold viruses—even though these viruses were trapped within cells. A 100% destruction is extremely potent and is unachieved by any drug.

For human infections this is a highly aggressive germicide. It is exceedingly powerful against molds and fungi. It is also highly destructive against viruses. There is a synergy from the combination of dessicated spice oils—wild oil of oregano, cumin oil, wild sage oil, and cinnamon oil. The drying of these oils into a powder concentrates their potency.

The dessicated multiple spice oil is found as capsules. This is the ideal form to use for difficult-to-resolve respiratory complaints, including tough cases of cold and flu. Thus, too, it is a powerful medicine for asthma and pneumonia.

How to take wild oregano

Without doubt, wild oregano is a strong substance. The extracts of this wild spice have a strong taste. They are also hot on both the tongue and taste buds. This heat largely explains the medicinal properties. Regardless, for some people this poses a challenge, that is for regular and daily consumption. So, it is a good idea to explain the various ways to consume this to improve compliance.

Sublingual versus oral

Oil of wild oregano made through steam distillation is the main wild oregano supplement. This is a highly powerful and versatile natural remedy. It is found in a dropper bottle consisting of the wild oregano oil emulsified in extra virgin olive oil. Ideally, this should be taken sublingually, that is under the tongue. It should not, however, be taken *on* the tongue, because, here, it creates too much sensation and burning. Regardless, sublingually, the absorption is rapid. Plus, this is the best way to take the oregano oil for conditions of the head and neck, for instance, sinus problems.

Yet, for some people because of the taste and heat this is impossible. This is despite the fact that this is temporary and the oil is rapidly absorbed into the body without any prolonged sensation. It is much more pleasant than, for instance, raw garlic or cayenne pepper.

So, the compliance for some people with the oil may not be ideal. The person may do it occasionally but never routinely. Thus, another option is to take it in water or juice. In particular, the oil blends well in tomato or V-8 juice. It also blends well in organic milk as well as carrot juice. Some people take it in orange or grapefruit juice. Another option is to simply add it to a small glass of water. In water, however, it tends to coat the glass, and so there is some loss here.

Regardless, the main issue is to take it regularly. So, a person must simply find the method that is best suited.

Yet another option is to take the oil in gelatin capsules. This is an easy way to achieve compliance. There is no taste involved. Plus, through this relatively large amounts of the oil can be taken—and it can be taken consistently in divided doses. The main benefits can still be achieved by taking the oil orally, as either gelatin capsules or drops in juice/water, although, perhaps, the most ideal method is to take it sublingually.

In enema water

The enema is one of the most powerful medicines known to the human race. This is an ideal way to administer natural medicines. Oil of wild oregano is highly suited for this administration, particularly the water soluble type, that is the mycelized version. This mixes thoroughly with the enema solution. Simply add ten drops of this water soluble wild oregano oil to an enema solution. Retain as long as possible. This will deliver this effective natural medicine right where it is direly needed. If the water soluble version is unavailable the regular type in extra virgin olive oil may be added, about five drops per enema solution.

Much disease is caused by disorders of the gut. The intestinal tract, including the colon, is readily infected by a host of organisms. These pathogens greatly weaken the immune system, ultimately leading to disease. The organisms, which cause chronic infection of the gut, include *Candida albicans*, *Mycobacterium tuberculosis*, mycoplasma, HIV, staph, parasites, H. pylori, hepatitis viruses, cytomegalovirus, and avian tuberculosis. The oregano-based enema solution is a direct means to purge the gut of these infections.

Topical scrubbing

This is a powerful method for using the oil of wild oregano as well as other heat-producing oils. The skin can essentially be scrubbed with oregano oil for profound effects.

There are a number of benefits from this method of administration. This by-passes the gut and, essentially, places the medicine directly into the body. This is because such heat-producing oils are readily absorbed by the lymph. It is the lymph which, then, carries the oil directly into the general circulation.

The lymph massage is highly invigorating. It is also medicinal, that is it is a technique that can be used in the treatment and reversal of disease. This can be applied along with the oral treatment. The scrubbing greatly stimulates the flow of lymph as well as blood. This helps stimulate the healing process. It is also a way of getting additional amounts of the oil of wild oregano into the bloodstream, so that this oil can act as a systemic antiseptic. Also, the scrubbing action helps activate the bone marrow and therefore this action stimulates the synthesis of white blood cells. This is particularly true when scrubbing the oil over the bone marrow sites, which are the shins, the top of the thigh bones (over the quadriceps muscles), the spinal column, and the sternum, that is the breast bone.

Foot massage

This is an exceptional means for the use of spice oils. Actually, spice oils are highly penetrating—the largest pores in the body are found on the soles of the feet. Scrubbing or rubbing the bottom of the feet is highly invigorating. This scrubbing leads to an increase lymph drainage as well as blood flow.

A vibrator may also be used. The oil may be rubbed into the soles of the feet and then the vibrator applied. This helps open up the pores and drives the oregano oil into the tissues. For infants and children foot massage is the ideal means of administration. This method may also be used for newborns. It is entirely safe to apply this in all such age categories. For sick infants/children the oil may be applied in this manner repeatedly, that is until the condition is resolved.

Foot soaking and ionic cleansing

Regarding the skin surface the feet have the largest pores in the body. The traditional regularly washing of the feet, practiced by early prophets and particularly by the Prophet Muhammad, may now largely be explained. This is how toxins can be purged from the body. These are toxins largely held within the lymphatic system as well as the blood and liver.

It is possible to take advantage of these pores through soaking therapies. Also, there are highly sophisticated foot baths, which create ionic charges for pulling poisons out of the body through the pores, located on the soles of the feet. For a simple foot soak use a basin filled with warm water or water as hot as can be tolerated. This helps enlarge the pores. Add per half gallon water a teaspoon of sea salt. Also, add 50 or more drops of water soluble, that is mycelized, oil of wild oregano. Or, add a tablespoon of emulsified multiple spice spray. Soak the feet for at least and hour, and repeat as often as needed.

Regarding the ionic foot baths this is a powerful system for detoxification. These units are now becoming readily available in naturally-inclined medical and health centers. When taking these ionic foot baths for multiplied benefit always add either the mycelized oil of oregano or the multiple spice spray.

Intranasal

Surely, the oil can be taken intranasally. However, this causes a significant amount of heat sensation and therefore discomfort. This discomfort is temporary. Even so, for both acute and chronic sinus conditions this is highly effective. An equally effective way is to spray the oil into the nose in the form of a sinus/nasal mist. This is a combination of the oil of wild oregano plus natural sea salt, along with oils of wild sage and bay leaf. With this water/saline based nasal spray there is some temporary burning. However, it is not near as severe as that experienced from taking the oil directly.

This is an important way to take the wild oregano. The sinuses house numerous pathogens. In particular, they house vile forms of fungi, which gain residence in this wet and dark environment. These fungi or rather molds cause great inflammation in the sinus cavities. Even so, this inflammation may extend into the Eustacion tube and from there the inner ear. In fact, the mold infection may become disseminated in this critical region. This can lead to ringing in the ear, disturbances in balance, that is vertigo, and ultimately deafness. All this is potentially reversible through using the wild oregano-based nasal spray, which will help root out the deep-seated fungal infestation in these regions. Such a spray is a potent cleansing agent, since the saline base assists in the penetration of the spice oils. Furthermore, saline has a direct tonic action upon the walls of the sinuses, while oils of wild oregano, bay leaf, and sage are highly antifungal, especially when absorbed into the mucous membranes.

The majority of people have deep-seated or hidden mold infections of the sinus cavities. According to a study done at Mayo Clinic (1999), mold infestation is the primary cause of chronic sinus conditions. In this study it was determined that when assessing 100 people with chronic sinusitis in all cases there was mold infection, while, incredibly, no evidence of a bacterial cause could be found. What's more, rather than merely one mold or fungus being causative in dozens of cases the individuals were infected with up to eight different molds. A wild oregano-based saline nasal solution is an effective means to eradicate such fungal infections. Such a solution should be used daily until the condition is normalized. This is used, along with the oil of oregano, which ideally should be taken sublingually.

Fungal infection and the power of wild oregano

Fungal infection is the bugaboo of human life. This is especially true of modern humans. A fungus is defined as a saprophyte, which means an organism that literally saps life. It even means an organism, which lives by taking life or rather lives on organisms which are dying. Webster's says that a saprophyte is an organism, which lives on "dead and decaying tissue." Then, for those humans who have fungal infections what does this imply about the state of their health? It is surely not very encouraging. Ultimately, it means that the persons are dying a slow death, while being eaten alive by the fungi.

This is surely a motive for killing these germs. Too, this would liberate the body and the immune system to better health. This is the benefit that the wild oregano achieves. There are other spice oils which do so. Sometimes it is beneficial to use them in combination. Of course, wild oregano is the main fungal killer. Yet, fungi are stubborn, so a multiple spice extract with synergistic powers may also be required. Other spice oils which are significantly antifungal include oil of wild bay leaf, oil of wild sage, oil of cumin, oil of wild myrtle, oil of allspice, oil of clove, and oil of cinnamon. Yet, even fruit, vegetable, and seed oils exert a degree of antifungal activity such as oils of black seed, avocado oil, extra virgin olive oil, primrose oil, crude cold pressed sesame oil, black currant seed oil, and sacha inchi oil. So, for a true antifungal diet such oils must be taken liberally. Yet, the real killers of fungi are the hot spicy oils, which have a noticeable heat and burning sensation.

New York City podiatrist Alexander Fish knows the nature of fungal infestation, since he sees this continuously. Fungi love to attack areas of poor or sluggish circulation such as the feet. Fish uses antifungal formulas based upon wild oregano, sage, and bay leaf. Such oils, he notes, have a power known as excoriation. This means, essentially, that the oils 'burn' or 'erode' the local tissues. This is invaluable, because this is how the oils assist in conquering the fungi by essentially rooting them out of the tissues and exposing them, then, killing them. Erosion, says Fish, is good. Without it, there would be no efficient way to kill the fungus. This is because the fungus is a deep-seated organism, in other words, it deeply invades tissue. So, the ideal natural medicine for eradicating it is somewhat aggressive, even slightly caustic, within the tissues. This describes spices oils, including oil of wild oregano, because these oils are highly aggressive. Despite this aggression, these spice oils are safe for human use. In other words, they have potent penetrating powers. This is a good property, since it is essential for the purging and destruction of invading fungi.

Fungi make life miserable. A person who feels awful, who is full of pain and stiffness—who suffers with exhaustion and constant sickness—such a person is likely overwhelmed by fungi. In addition, those with muscular disorders are often fungally contaminated. The same is true of people with mental diseases. Frequently, with such syndromes fungi are a major culprit. This is because fungi produce poisons, which contaminate the nervous system as well as the muscles and joints.

In the Western world there are countless millions of people who suffer from fungal infestation. This is a consequence of modern living. It is also a consequence of the typical food available in Western civilization. Too, it is the results of the types of drugs commonly prescribed, in particular, antibiotics.

As mentioned previously these fungi are deep-seated invaders. Normally, they rarely invade the tissue. This only happens after the tissues break down or there is a collapse of the immune system. Also, numerous man-made substances cause fungal overgrowth and therefore invasion. Chief among these is refined sugar, which plays an enormous role in fungal overload. So does the overuse of antibiotics rather any antibiotic use. Yes it is true, even a single course of antibiotics may result in fungal invasion. Imagine the status of those who consume vast quantities of antibiotics, repeated doses. Such individuals are completely infested by fungi, which have invaded virtually all recesses of their bodies.

Know this: fungi can invade every part of the body. This is true even of the brain and spinal cord. Moreover, this is a common consequence of the massive use of antibiotics. Of course, this is because such antibiotics destroy the healthy bacteria. It is the healthy bacteria, which are the body's defense against fungal invasion. When they are decimated, then, the fungi has free reign to devastate the tissues. It does so by vigorously invading, first, the mucous membranes. These are the membranes, which line the mouth, sinuses, bronchial tubes, esophagus, intestines, vagina, bladder, and urethra. All such regions are vulnerable for attack by fungi, especially after a course or two of antibiotics.

Antibiotics are a great perpetrator of deep seated infections. They drive the fungus into deepest recesses of the body. Then, these organisms become firmly established and are, therefore, difficult to eradicate. Thus, surely, drugs and chemical antibiotics are the major cause of resistant fungal infections.

Then, the degree of the infection is dependent upon the degree of the intake of antibiotics. A few courses of these drugs will surely cause chronic fungal infection. Yet, numerous or dozens of courses will cause extreme fungal infestation.

If anyone is sick, they should consider a few simple issues. Is the sick person a recipient of numerous doses of antibiotics. This should be carefully assessed. Also, is the person a sugar addict, or was such a one a sugar addict in the past? Or, has the person been on steroids for a prolonged period, now or in the past?

There is another factor which must be considered. This relates to where a person lives. If a person lives in an area of great moisture and humidity, then the likelihood of fungal infestation is high. The home or work is also worth considering. Could there possibly be mold contamination in the building, either now or in the past, which could have exposed the sick person to a strain or several strains of killer molds? Could, then, those molds have colonized such a person's body?

Everyone knows from toenail fungus that mold/fungal infections are stubborn. There is no way for the body on its own to clear the infection. Once this infection becomes established it is there virtually permanently, that is unless it is aggressively treated with special medicines. Even then, even when taking the most potent antifungal drugs known, the infection usually returns.

How can such a pathogen exist, which can overwhelm all human defenses? In fact, it makes sense that this pathogen can do so, since it has been in existence for countless billions of years. Long before there were humans fungi were well established. Their purpose has always been to degrade matter: to thrive off of dead or dying material, including a damaged or weakened human body. So, a fungus has powers greater than the most potent human powers. It knows what to do to survive better than does the human organism.

Fungi have a number of unique means to ensure their survival. One such means is deep invasion of the tissues. Fungi are experts at this. By this they can become well established in their victims. This invasion is partly the result of enzymes, which the fungi produce in order to digest tissue. It is also mechanical, since these organisms produce a kind of tentacle, which has invasive powers. Also, the fungi attempt to neutralize the immune system. They do so also by producing, incredibly, fungal toxins which directly poison immune cells. Fungi also achieve an action, which is highly dangerous. They actually invade the cells and attempt to overrun the human genetic material. It is now known that invasive fungi take over the genetic powers of human cells by splicing in their own genetic code, causing the cells to function, essentially, for the fungi instead of the actual human. Thus, through stealth the fungi blend themselves into the human organism, as if they are one. Through this these invaders effectively neutralize all immune response. This is why the cure must come from an outside power. This is the power of wild oregano and other potent antifungal spice extracts.

It is not always obvious that there is fungal infection. There may not be a specific blood test that reveals it. Nor are there always obvious symptoms, which are definitive. Nor can it be necessarily revealed that there is obvious fungus growing on or in the body. Scans and scopes do not usually reveal it. Nor do x-rays. This infection must be largely presumed based upon the history and symptoms. This is true even if the symptoms are vague.

Remember, fungi are stealth invaders. They do not want to make themselves known. So, they have a number of devices for remaining hidden. By the time people know about them they have already severely invaded the tissues. They have already developed their home.

Fungal infection: a major cause of disease

So, how does a person know that he/she has fungus in the body, that is the type which invades the tissues and causes disease? It is relatively easy to determine. Anyone who has had a prolonged course of antibiotics, two weeks or more, has some degree of fungal invasion. Taking antibiotics continuously for three or more weeks assures the infection.

Yet, anyone who has repeatedly taken these drugs, course upon course over a period of months or years, definitely has fungal infection of a most profound type. This is true, even if no obvious symptoms exist. There may be toenail fungus, athlete's foot, occasional fatigue, and no other symptoms and still the infection is severe. It is merely hidden. Yet, left untreated there may be serious consequences, including life-threatening diseases such as cancer, arthritis, stroke, diabetes, and heart disease.

Definitely, fungal infection is associated with all such diseases. Allowing the infection to fester in the body without taking action is a disaster. It is only a matter of time before the tissues are consumed and terminal disease results. Yet, this is all avoidable by taking aggressive action against the fungus or fungi. This is through the potent antifungal power of spice oils, particularly oil of wild oregano, oil of wild sage, oil of cumin, and oil of bay leaf. The point is if the fungi are allowed to continuously invade the body, they will eventually cause disease. Thus, to prevent such disease or to reverse existing disease these fungi must be killed.

There are diseases which tell of the existence of fungal infection. If a person has such a disease or diseases, then, the likelihood is exceedingly high that fungal invasion is the cause or at least a major part of this cause. These diseases directly correlated with fungal invasion include diabetes, cancer, heart disease, scleroderma, stroke, lupus, fibromyalgia, and arthritis. There are dozens of other diseases which have a massive fungal connection. These diseases are wrongly deemed inflammatory disorders, while, in fact, they are infectious diseases—and it is the infection, which leads to inflammation. In this regard the fungi play a monumental role. In certain of these disease fungi play the primary role. These diseases include Sjogren's syndrome (dry eye sicca), ulcerative colitis, Crohn's disease, sinusitis, allergic rhinitis, bronchitis, asthma, ankylosing spondylitis, autoimmune thyroiditis (Hashimoto's disease), and Addison's diseases. Incredibly, when the fungal infections within the body are cleared, usually these diseases are reversed.

Even mental disorders may be caused by fungi. Again, fungi produce toxins, which can poison the cells. This includes the cells of the nervous system. It is now known that fungal toxins are a cause of a wide range of mental disorders, including depression, anxiety, and even insanity. For instance, the insane behavior of the people of Salem, which led to the Salem Witch Trials, was due to a fungal toxin, in this case ergotamine, a poison that resulted from moldy rye. The insane behavior of the people was strictly because of the hallucinogenic effects of ergotamine, which is similar chemically to LSD. Thus, mental instability may be caused by fungi as the main perpetrator.

Mental, neurological, and psychological diseases which may be caused by fungal infection include Alzheimer's disease, Parkinson's disease, multiple sclerosis, schizophrenia, manic-depressive syndrome, anxiety neurosis, mental retardation, autism, and attention deficit disorder. Incredibly, in many instances when the fungal infections are cleared people with these conditions improve dramatically.

It is well known that, acutely, fungi can infect the spinal cord and brain. What is less well known is that these organisms can also do so chronically. Furthermore, it is usually forgotten that the fungal toxins alone are sufficient to cause diseases of the nervous system, brain, and spinal cord, including frank mental/psychological diseases. Fungal toxins are highly poisonous to the nerves and brain. In infinitesimal quantities they can poison the entire nervous system. A simple approach to nerve and brain diseases is to merely take the antifungal spice treatment for a week or so. This would be mainly the oil of wild oregano plus the dessicated multiple spice oil complex. Also, as a means to gain wild oxygenated compounds for the brain the oregano juice may also be taken. If improvement is noted, then, the fungal role is confirmed.

Again, for severe afflictions of the brain the juice is essential. This juice is actually a steam extract, where the steam interacts with the oregano to form a watery extract. Unlike the oil this watery extract or juice readily dissolves into the brain and other nerve tissue, including the spinal cord. Here, it can help purge the nervous system of any infectious invaders, including molds, fungi bacteria, and viruses.

It must always be remembered that rather than the cause of sudden, that is acute, illnesses fungi invade mainly chronically. These organisms establish themselves to parasitize the host. Thus, they seek a mutually beneficial relationship. Ideally, for the fungus it is best merely to erode the host, not destroy it. What's more, because of this chronic nature of the various fungal infections it is not easy to eradicate them. To do so requires a major effort, and the treatment must be consistent. This is the only way to guarantee the destruction of these pathogens.

Yet, it is not just the nervous system which is affected. In chronic fungal invasion virtually all organs are infected. In some cases all cells in the body may be invaded by these aggressors. This causes extreme toxicity and, ultimately, fatality.

The fungi must be vigorously destroyed. Also, the various fungal toxins must be purged. Regarding the destruction of the fungi only the spice oils are capable of achieving this. These oils may be taken either sublingually or orally and also rubbed topically. In some cases these oils may be applied vaginally and also rectally. This is particularly true of the less heat-producing oils such as oil of wild bay leaf, oil of wild sage, and oil of cumin. Even so, certainly, all such oils must be in an extra virgin olive oil base before being applied to or in sensitive regions such as the genitals and rectum.

Yet, the main treatment is orally, either as drops under the tongue or by mouth (that is swallowed). For best results both drops under the tongue and oral doses should be taken. The mainstay of treatment is the wild oil in extra virgin olive oil—be sure to procure this from a reputable manufacturer, which has done research—and the multiple spice complex, which consists of dessicated wild spice oils in capsule form. This may be supported by the crude herb/*Rhus coriaria* combination as well as the wild oregano juice.

The supportive phase of treatment is to apply the oil topically. This is by scrubbing it into the soles of the feet, along the shins, up and down the tops and sides of the thighs, and possibly about the clavicles and sternum (that is breast bone). The latter regions are areas of great lymphatic reflexes, in fact, this is where the lymphatic fluid dumps into the general circulation.

Yet another method of treatment is vaginal or rectal insertion. This cannot be done with the oil of wild oregano (when diluted, the high grade brand is safe for this purpose) unless it is diluted in additional extra virgin olive oil. This is through taking the existing bottle, which is already emulsified in extra virgin olive oil and diluting this 10 to 1. This will reduce the burning sensation to a tolerable level, even though when using the undiluted form this sensation, while extreme, is temporary. Again, as mentioned previously there are other oils which can be applied in these regions that do not burn. These oils include oils of wild bay leaf, sage, and myrtle as well as oil of cumin.

Chapter Two

Colds and Flu: Oregano to the Rescue

Colds and flu are no contest to the powers of wild oregano extracts. Yet, these are illnesses for which modern medicine has no cure. It is incredible that in all modern medicine there are no cures for these plagues. Drugs only treat symptoms. Even so, some of these drugs, such as those which suppress fever and coughs, may actually prolong the illness.

Are vaccines any better? According to a study by Lone Simonson, 2007, of the U. S. Government's National Institutes of Health (NIH) for the elderly the flu vaccine 'doesn't have any effect.' Simonson established that there is no scientific proof, in fact, not even a single reputible scientific study proving the shot's efficacy, paticularly in people over 70. In other words, through taking the vaccine there is no improvement in either the incidence of this disease or the symptoms. This is bizarre. Why would the medical system promote a treatment, which is useless? Too, why would the people subject themselves to this for no reason? Perhaps fear of death alone is sufficient reason to undergo bizarre treatments, which have no beneficial effects.

The flu vaccine is useless. It doesn't kill the virus or viruses. Regardless, each year there are dozens of strains of flu viruses. A vaccine would merely be a guess, covering, perhaps, two or three strains. Must medicine be based merely on guesswork? Surely, this doesn't add to the credibility of its approach. Then, the accuracy of Simonson's government-sponsored study is obvious. This is because it is worse than useless. The debacle of this vaccine is even more extreme than its mere uselessness. As demonstrated by Simonson people who took the vaccine fared worse than those who refused it. Incredibly, in vaccine takers the death rate was significantly higher than those who avoided the shot. Thus, said Simonson, the claim for the vaccine to have any use in saving lives is preposterous.

In contrast, with extracts of wild oregano there is no guesswork. It is a potent antiviral agent. It is also a powerful antifungal agent, which finds immense utility versus colds, since many cold syndromes are caused by molds.

Colds and flu are associated with the build-up of mucous. Wild oregano, particularly the steam-extracted oil, is a potent mucolytic agent, which means it breaks apart and thins mucous. With flu in particular irritating or even severe coughs may be associated, especially in post flu syndrome. Again, wild oregano comes to the rescue, since it is one of the most powerful antitussive agents known, which means it halts cough.

The mechanism against cough is different than drugs. Rather than suppressing the cough through chemical antagonists the wild oregano attacks the root of the cough, which is the irritant. It destroys and cleanses such irritants, also dissolving any obstructions. Thus, it offers a healthy mechanism for eliminating this symptom. There is no need to cough once the irritant is purged.

Regarding the flu there are a number of other distressing symptoms with this syndrome. One of them is weakness and prostration. This is because of toxins produced in the body by the invaders. It is also because of the toxins the body produces in the attempt to destroy these invaders. All these toxins are neutralized by the wild oregano.

Some of these toxins are highly potent. This is no matter. The wild oregano, particularly the steam distilled oil as drops under the tongue, has a direct antitoxic action against these poisons. This is true of any microbial poison, even the highly potent and potentially fatal staphylococcal endotoxin and the clostridial botulism toxin.

Even so, the real power of the wild oregano is easy to realize. It is a power that no drug can match. This is the power of the destruction of the actual cold and flu viruses. This is a destruction which has been confirmed by scientific studies. The first hint of the mechanism behind its extensive antiviral powers was determined by Siddiqui and colleagues publishing in *Medical Science Research.* Here, it was found that the wild oregano oil destroyed a variety of cold and flu viruses, as well as herpes-like viruses. In fact, noted the researchers, the viruses were "disintegrated" by the oil.

The most extensive research, however, was performed by Ijaz and Ingram at Microbiotest. In a high quality assessment in tissue culture the wild oregano oil from the Mediterranean spice proved exceedingly powerful. This oil destroyed both cold and flu viruses and even destroyed at a higher dose the bird flu virus. An abstract showing the findings was presented at the Seventeenth International Conference on Antiviral Research in Tucson, Arizona (2004). Attending were a number of representatives of the pharmaceutical industry. These representatives, noted the presenter, were visibly shocked by the findings, since they had never before seen such compelling results. In other words, the drug company representatives realized that no drug in existence could match the virus-killing powers of this impressive substance.

No wonder the wild oregano extracts are so popular. People have found them to be effective for conditions for which there are no medical cures. For decades in the Western world a deliberate cure has been sought for these conditions. Now that cure has been found, moreover, there is no doubt about its effectiveness. Its power has been proven in lab studies, and it has passed the test of time, being used by countless societies for centuries. For colds/flu the ancient Egyptians, Greeks, Hittites, Sumerians, Babylonians, Romans, and Islaamic peoples all used it. Moreover, it was used extensively in medieval Europe for colds, flu, and earaches as well as pneumonia, asthma, and bronchitis.

So, again, its effectiveness against such minor germs is well demonstrated. This is because for the wild oregano the destruction of cold and flu viruses is no issue, since this oil is capable of destroying far more noxious germs, such as pseudomonas, staph, strep, clostridium, klebsiella, proteus, and candida, than mere viruses. It was merely an additional proof to show it in the laboratory, that is to prove its powers directly.

At Microbiotest, the testing method which was used is known as in vitro, which means outside a living body. However, the technique is impressive, since the virus is actually grown in living cells, which are cultured and then incubated in a nutrient broth. So, again, the virus is within the cells, infecting and killing them.

Then, the wild oil of oregano was added to the culture medium. As a result, the viruses were destroyed. With the cold and flu virus, in this case the human corona virus, the oil of wild oregano achieved a 99.9% destruction, while the multiple spice extract proved superior, killing 100% of all organisms. This included the various pathogens lodged deep within the tissue culture cells. Thus, the oregano oil proved to be an intracellular germicide. Notably, it achieves the same effect within human cells. With the flu virus, that is influenza, similar results were obtained. The flu is a more dire illness than colds; the virus is more difficult to kill. Thus, using a dose ten times greater than used for the cold virus similar results were achieved, that is a 99.7% kill. This, too, was in tissue culture. The bird flu virus was also killed, although the dosage necessary was massive, some 25 times greater than that used to kill the human flu virus. In both cases, that is the human flu and the bird flu, the multiple spice extract proved most powerful, killing more viruses more vigorously and quickly. This multiple spice extract consists of dessicated wild oils of oregano and sage, along with dessicated oils of cumin and cinnamon. This is an exceedingly powerful formula for use in tough or resistant infections, although it is safe to take daily in modest amounts such as a capsule or two daily. Truly, as proven by scientific studies the multiple spice extract is the most powerful type of wild oregano or spice supplement known.

Even so, there is virtually no information about wild oregano or similar potent spices in herbal books, that is those books which describe herbal medicines. In fact, regarding the powers and uses of wild oregano there is more information in this book than, surely, all other books on herbal or natural medicine in existence. Yet, this neglect of the subject is strictly modern.

There was significant mention of the greatness of wild oregano, as well as similar antiseptic spices, such as wild sage, cumin, cinnamon, and wild bay leaf, in earlier books. In the 1500s through 1600s British and Irish herbalists gave significant mention of these spices, describing them as indispensable medicines. Here, the spices and their extracts were held as cures for a wide range of disorders, including diarrhea, stomach conditions, earaches, colds, flu, rhinitis, and infected wounds. With rare exceptions no such mention of this benefit of spices is found in modern texts. Yet, in ancient Rome cinnamon, a powerful antiseptic and preservative, was bought for an equal weight of gold. Moreover, early British herbalists, including Culpepper, Salmon, and Gerard, gave much praise to wild oregano for its effectiveness against infectious diseases, particularly head colds, lung infections, and earaches.

Culpepper's 17th century writings alone demonstrate the real power of this spice-medicine. Despite the huge number of herbs he commends he states that wild oregano reigns supreme in a number of illnesses. According to Culpepper the illnesses for which oregano is the top natural medicine include food poisoning (sour stomach), head congestion/colds, cough (and, therefore lung infections) intestinal disorders, stomachache, gastric disorders, tuberculosis, hepatitis, and ear disorders. Salmon, who wrote in the 1500s, agrees, essentially saying that there is for numerous illnesses no natural medicine superior to wild oregano and that the oil in particular is a categorical cure for head and neck disorders, including colds and earaches.

There is no reason to diminish the importance of such early findings. People then were highly learned. Many people were scholars in numerous fields. Surely, their observations are trustworthy. Moreover, they deemed substances cures because of the specific results they achieved. Drugs, they knew, not only failed to be curative, but they also usually made the patient more ill or even caused fatality.

In the early 1900s in the United States there were a number of books published on natural medicine. In these books a variety of therapies were described. Virtually all the prescribed therapies were natural, although, admittedly some of the natural substances, such as mercurial and arsenical compounds, are themselves poisonous. Yet, what is most revealing is the titles they used to describe these treatments. In the *Library of Health*, published in the 1920s, there is an entire section titled Curative Medicine. Curiously, this was written before the establishment of drug monopolies by the petrochemical cartel. The cures which are described included essential oils, boric acid, hot baths, roots, and herbs as well as a certain amount of drugs. Yet, the point is all such substances were listed as curative. In other words, there was no attempt to diminish the natural substances, to belittle them, saying they are "unproven." Nor was it claimed that they were ineffective.

The government says this is not so. Natural substances, it proclaims, have no curative properties, and their popular use necessitates laboratory science to prove any effect. This is the opposite of the statements of countless thousands of researchers and practitioners, who have used natural medicines from the beginnings of civilization. Again, countless millions of people have established the curative powers of nature. The various peoples from antiquity to early modern times saw herbal medicines as a proven therapy. Plus, modern research proves the vast power of natural substances. Yet, what evidence does the government have to dispute it? There is no such evidence. On the contrary the evidence in the government's possession confirms these earlier and even ancient findings. Regardless, it isn't the government which disputes it. Rather, it is the people who are the powers behind the government who are responsible. For them natural medicine is a monumental threat. This is because the use of such medicine erodes at the profits of such individuals, that is the supremely wealthy ones, who control the government.

So, any belittlement of natural medicine is merely a plot. This plot is for the maintenance of the monopoly to control the flow of wealth. It has nothing to do with the legitimacy of natural medicine. That was already established long ago. After all, it was the great scriptures which gave guidance to the human race. Here, the people are told of the greatness of the divine medicines—and these foods/herbs are called medicines and cures. The Bible tells all people to purge with wild oregano, while the Qur'aan deems natural honey a legitimate medicine, a "blessing for all humankind." Both the Qur'aan and the Bible mention herbage, most likely wild herbage, as a blessing and benefit for the human race. Is the government, now, seeking to regulate the divine word? If so, this entity will never achieve it. Nature will always provide, and the human being can always harvest its goods. No one can stop people from taking advantage of wild nature.

The powers of wild oregano are undeniable. Today, it works equally as well as stated by early scholars. The cold virus is no match for wild oregano, particularly the steam extracted oil. The flu virus also succumbs, but this may require larger and more frequent doses. Regarding potentially devastating flu viruses, which may cause pandemics, these, too, succumb, yet, again, even larger doses are required. In contrast, there are no synthetic substances—no drugs—which offer any such powers.

Can anyone imagine it? Is there a drug that has more than one power, which can reverse two diseases? Imagine a drug which can reverse not merely two but, rather, countless diseases. This is the wild oregano, the powers of which are vast and which have been proven by the test of time.

A person gets a cold. The Mediterranean-source hand-picked wild oregano oil is used as drops under the tongue. The dosage is about three to five drops every fifteen minutes or, perhaps, half hour. The cold is obliterated within the hour or at most within the day. Is this not an absolute cure? There are people who eliminate their colds with one or two doses. No one can argue the power of such a substance, which naturally and safely reverses disease. Yet, these are diseases for which modern medicine offers no cure.

A person contracts the flu. The true Mediterranean spice-based oil of wild oregano is consumed as drops under the tongue, five or more drops every fifteen minutes, half hour, or hour. The multiple spice capsule is also consumed, two capsules every hour or every two hours. The flu syndrome is halted within an hour, a few hours, or at most within a day or two. Thus, the wild oregano and multiple spice extract safely and powerfully reverse a dreaded syndrome. Yet, no medicine of any kind can do so, nor could entire categories of such medicines do so. Skeptics should try it. Then, they will be convinced. As a result, they will never use any other therapy for colds and flu, as well as earaches, bronchitis, and cough, other than the wild oregano.

So, then, the wild oregano extracts, as well as extracts of other spices, are cures for colds and flu. These extracts obliterate all such viruses. Can there be any other conclusion?

Chapter Three

Saving Lives:
The Case Histories

Wild oregano is the most powerful herb known. This power is particularly critical regarding the immune system. It protects and strengthens the immune system, while also killing noxious germs. Then, in fact, germs are a major cause of illness.

To reverse serious diseases people need such power. When they discover it and all that it can do for their health, then, they realize its greatness. All the skepticism/resistance is eliminated. These are people who may have tried any number of remedies for their ailments, largely to no avail. Then, suddenly, they discover the wild oregano. Then, in fact, they gain relief. They may even achieve an absolute cure, while no other therapy did so. This often leads to much gratitude and even tears.

Here, people are largely shocked. They are astonished at the fact that this natural medicine alone reversed their disorders. Thus, they gratefully give testimony of the result. This section includes real case histories of actual people who greatly benefitted, who know that wild oregano and other spice extracts are precisely the cause for their improvement and even for their cure.

Even so, there is great resistance against oregano's power. This resistance is because of vested interests. Such a simple natural substance truly threatens powerful business concerns. People who rely upon the wild oregano no longer need drugs. They greatly reduce their use of drugs or eliminate them completely. This is why it is resisted and/or attacked.

Regardless, rather than a drug wild oregano is a natural medicine. It contains a wide range of medicinal compounds, including phenols, polyphenols, flavonoids, terpenes, long chain alcohols, esters, and in the case of the whole crude herb trace minerals as well as phytosterols. All such substances have positive/medicinal actions on the body. Thus, the only consequence is that wild oregano will help the health, nothing derogatory.

People rave about the benefits of wild oregano as well as other potent spices. In particular, there are countless reports regarding the powers of the extracts of wild oregano, particularly the oil. These reports are highly revealing, because they are real—because they are compelling evidence of the ultimate benefits. A specific result which a person derives has meaning, in many ways just as much as a scientific study. In fact, this is scientific. If a person takes the wild oregano, for instance, for a sinus infection and/or bronchial condition and, then, it works virtually immediately, this is invaluable information. It tends to prove that the wild oregano has great powers for the mucous membranes of the respiratory tract. It also tells that this is a potent antihistaminic agent as well as a power germ-killer.

When people say that the oregano oil gives them relief for their sinus/bronchial conditions virtually immediately, it is like a study unto itself, because it proves that these conditions must be caused by mucous membrane infection or at a minimum irritation of the membranes from toxins. This is because the wild oregano oil is both a broad spectrum germicide as well as an antidote to toxic irritants such as mycotoxins, pollens, and noxious chemicals, all of which readily induce inflammation in the respiratory tract. Thus, no one must belittle the case histories. They are a gold mine of information which reveal the real causes of diseases as well as the cures.

People give amazing testimonies regarding the powers of wild oregano. This is because they are often desperate and have tried numerous therapies to no avail. So, they are willing to volunteer the precise results with great vigor. It is noticeable, since for most people the orthodox therapies have proven inadequate and in many cases noxious. Then, the wild oregano treatment produces deliberate results, that is massive improvement occurs, and there can be no doubt about it.

Even so, there will be dissenters. Safe, natural treatments are a threat to many financial interests. Here, there will be an attempt to denigrate these cases—these true reports of the people—as "unscientific." The dissenters may even claim the case histories as fraudulent. Yet, make no mistake about it these are true stories, which are reported directly from the people. In fact, a conservative approach is taken with these examples to ensure accuracy. What follows is real and can be used as examples for those who are suffering from various diseases. So, take advantage of the information. It may well prove invaluable in a person's search for answers—for actual cures—against health crises of all types as well as degenerative diseases.

Regardless, there is no claim to cure for the various human diseases. Rather, it is merely a statement of fact, of actual human experience will likely prove invaluable to another person in need. That is the purpose of the following testimonials. It is to truly help the fellow human in the search for assistance and cure. This is the true purpose of the medical profession. What's more, all of them are true, and thus if a person is afflicted with a similar disease as those included in the testimonials, he/she should expect the same positive and dramatic results. Included are testimonials of adults and children, as well as infants and pets, as follows:

Man with persistent asthma cured with oil of wild oregano plus dessicated multiple spice capsules

Mr. N. is a 50-year-old man who developed persistent asthma. The condition was marked by significant inflammation in the bronchial tubes. He was taking bronchodialators and steroids, to no avail. Oil of oregano and dessicated wild multiple spice capsules were recommended to him. He took them, and, astonishingly, the inflammation and breathing difficulty were rapidly eliminated. Within three days he achieved complete relief rather eradication of all symptoms. The inflammation was eliminated. The cause, he said, was mold infection, and he reasoned, correctly, that the wild oregano and multiple spice extract obliterated the mold infestation. Once the infestation was eliminated the irritation was ceased, and, thus, the asthma was reversed.

Woman with yeast vaginitis cured with oil of wild oregano

Ms. R. is a 42-year-old woman with a predilection for sugar. She has a fetish for chocolate, plus she has used antibiotics repeatedly over the years. Suddenly, she developed a vaginal yeast infection. It was a moderate infection with itching and drainage. Then, she took several courses of antibiotics and it worsened, the vaginal walls becoming intensely red and inflamed. The itching was unbearable.

A course of wild oregano was begun using a super-powerful strength (triple strength) oil of wild oregano in extra virgin olive oil as sublingual drops. She took twenty drops twice daily. Within two weeks on this dosage, the infection was eradicated.

Headache in midst of a lecture eliminated

Ms. N. is a 50-year-old woman who suffers from regular migraines. She interrupted a lecture I was giving to complain about her migraine pain. I passed over to her a bottle of oil of wild oregano (regular strength, Mediterranean hand-picked) and instructed her to take several drops every five or ten minutes. After doing so, she exclaimed, the headache/migraine was gone. This dramatic result occurred in less than 30 minutes.

Ms. S, manager of Irish health food store chain, cured of potentially fatal condition in less than an hour

Ms. S. is a 43-year-old woman who was suffering from a dire circumstance. She had developed a potentially fatal form of diarrhea known as *Clostridium difficle*, which she contracted in a hospital. This was causing her to have bouts of diarrhea every five or ten minutes. Untreated, this could lead to colon resection and perhaps fatality.

Attending my lecture on behalf of her stores she sat at the back of the room for obvious reasons. When I found out her plight, I instructed her to take the oil of wild oregano (blue label brand) as drops under the tongue every five minutes, as much as 20 drops at a time. After doing so the entire condition was resolved. Incredibly, she was able to sit through the entire lecture/seminar, which lasted over two hours. Since then, she has recommended the wild oil to virtually all her customers.

Potentially fatal staph infection of the leg resolved within a week

Mr. C., a 75-year-old British man, suffered from the highly dire MRSA infection, which afflicted his lower leg. This drug-resistant staph attacked a wound in his lower leg, the wound being a consequence of diabetes. The high (super) strength version of the wild oil of oregano was applied. Wound healing was initiated virtually immediately. What's more, all serious symptoms of pain, throbbing, and inflammation were eliminated in less than a week. Mr. C. regarded this as a miracle, as should anyone, since this condition is incurable through modern medicine.

Tapeworm expelled by crude wild oregano herb combined with *Rhus coriaria*

Ms. T. is a 23-year-old worker at a health food store. Tall, she tends towards being thin. Feeling she needed to do a cleanse she fasted, drinking only sips of juice, while taking large amounts of the crude wild oregano plus rhus, garlic, and onion in capsule form (about nine capsules daily). After four days she expelled a three foot-long tapeworm. This she attributed exclusively to the wild crude oregano/rhus combination.

Severe leg cramp/spasm halted by wild oregano crude herbal capsules

Mr. B. is a 59-year-old worker in a nutritional company. Despite working in such an environment his diet is poor, as he eats processed foods. Occasionally, he gets night cramps in his legs and feet. While I visited Mr. B. he suffered a sudden onset of severe cramps in his calf muscle. I gave him the wild oregano crude herb in a capsule form with Rhus coriaria. Within five minutes he experienced significant relief, and within ten minutes the pain/cramping was completely gone. He no longer gets such cramps as long as he takes the wild oregano/rhus capsules.

Wild oregano has properties for relieving spasms and cramps. This may be due to the pain-relieving properties of its aromatic oils, but it is also related to the dense content of calcium, magnesium, and phosphorus in this herb. This may explain the dramatic results experienced by Mr. B.

A single one-ounce bottle of high strength oil of wild oregano obliterates chronic sinus infection in two weeks

Ms. T. is a 40-year-old woman with a history of a chronic sinus infection. She has had the infection for over five years. When the infection was severe, her sinuses would bleed. Ms. T. heard about the power of wild oregano oil and so bought a bottle of the oil, being instructed to take it vigorously. She took 20 to 40 drops three times daily sublingually. Within six hours the bleeding halted. Furthermore, after only 30 doses the sinus infection was eliminated. Simultaneously, she noted, a chronic vaginal yeast disorder was cured. This was the only 'side effect' she experienced.

Wild oregano extract, as a liquid steam-distilled juice, eradicates stomach tumor

Mrs. J. is a 60-year-old woman with a history of stomach cancer, as proven by CT scan. A non-surgical case all the medical therapies had failed. She was essentially sent home to die.

A famous maker of wild oregano products sent her at no-charge a gallon of wild oregano juice, along with the juice of wild rosemary. Both are steam-distilled extracts. She took both extracts at a dosage of a quarter cup of each daily. Thirty days later she had another CT scan. The tumor was eradicated.

Woman with serious so-called autoimmune disorder greatly aided by oil of wild oregano

Ms. O. suffered from a bizarre condition, known as Sjogren's syndrome, where her eyes were totally dry. This is also known as dry eye sicca. She began taking the oil of oregano in large amounts, about 60 drops (two droppersful) two or three times daily. She took bottles of the oil repeatedly, noticing improvement in a wide range of health conditions, including chronic fungal infections of the respiratory tract. After the seventeenth bottle, she said, "I noticed an amazing improvement with my dry eye syndrome..." Because the eyes were so dry, she couldn't live normally. She was unable to go out in the sun or go outdoors on windy days. However, after the aggressive oregano oil therapy she "could go outside in the sun" freely.

Infected knee in seven-year-old girl cured with oil of wild oregano (as reported by her mother, J.C.)

A seven-year-old girl scraped her knee, which then became infected. Antibiotic treatment was of no avail.

Ultimately, a bizarre growth developed over the site of injury, most likely a fungus. This became a chronic infection, which looked like a cross between a massive wart and a fungal infection. Doctors had no clue regarding the cause, and all medical treatments were useless. The mother, then, bought the oil of wild oregano and applied it. She simply dressed her daughter's lesion with an oregano oil dressing. Within two weeks this impossible infection was eliminated, exclusively because of the Mediterranean-source oil of wild oregano.

Wild oregano oil-based nasal spray with sage and bay leaf restores hearing in the permanently disabled.

Ms. C. is a 60-year-old woman with a history of deafness. The deafness apparently developed after several bouts of respiratory infections. Her physician said her hearing would never return, but she rejected this, reasoning that the cause was chronic infection. She religiously took a wild oregano oil-based nasal spray, made also with wild bay leaf and sage oils as well as sea salt. After three months of the daily use of this spray virtually all her hearing returned. This is a remarkable result and is surely a consequence of the antiseptic power of the spice oils, which were directly applied on the site of infection, clearing the ear (eustachian tube) passages, so hearing could be restored.

Chernobyl victim enjoys massive benefits from taking wild oregano juice and oil of wild oregano

Mrs. B. is a survivor of the Chernobyl disaster. However, her exposure left her sickened with a wide range of diseases, including massive fungal infestation and brain lesions. For Mrs. B. the diagnosis of Cushing's disease was made as well as a brain tumor. Religiously, she took the wild oregano, along with wild greens flush, undiluted royal jelly, and the juice of oregano. Three months after beginning this treatment Mrs. B. went to a research institute in Boston, Massachusetts, for follow-up in her treatment. Her doctors stated that her Cushing's disease had later "disappeared." In addition, some three years an MRI proved that her brain tumor had "shrunk considerably."

Woman with COPD who was on oxygen improves dramatically

Ms. W. had a condition known as COPD, which stands for chronic obstructive lung disease. The condition was so severe that she was on oxygen daily. After hearing that the wild oregano was good for the lungs she tried it. "It was the best thing," she said, "that ever happened to me." She also noted, incredibly, "It started improving my breathing immediately," and that she, as a result, was "now off all oxygen and can function normally…" This was an incredible result for a person who was in such a dire condition.

Tiny amount of oil of wild oregano, blue-label brand, obliterates cold

Mr. A. had a terrible cold, which lasted for three weeks. He coughed terribly and suffered from congestion. His wife, a big believer in oil of oregano, talked him into taking it at a dosage of two drops under the tongue twice daily. In three days as reported by his wife the cold was gone. What's more, he experienced the 'side effect' of a great boost in energy.

Sinus surgery avoided through the use of wild oregano oil

Mr. L. suffered from a severe chronic sinus infection. After over a year of treatment with potent drugs to no avail he was given the only option, which was surgery. His symptoms were constant mucous drainage, post nasal drip, a reduction in hearing, ringing in the ear, and a foul smell from the nose.

He was placed on the oil of wild oregano and the multiple spice dessicated capsules made from wild oregano oil, wild sage oil, cumin oil, and cinnamon oil. Within three months he was "symptom free." During that time, however, his doctor kept calling him, saying that he must schedule for surgery or he would be "in trouble." These pressure tactics did not deter him, and he kept to the therapy relentlessly.

Mr. L. suffered only two side effects. These were an improvement in both his toenails and fingernails, which were infected by fungi.

Woman on narcotics given relief through wild spices

Mrs. B. is a 50-year-old woman who suffers from terminal pain due to broken bones and arthritis. In what was an incredible response she saw massive relief of her pain by taking a combination of oil of wild oregano with the multiple spice dessicated extract. She was able to halt the narcotics and simply uses the wild oregano and multiple spice extracts for the pain. This is a major achievement, considering the addictive nature of these drugs.

6% essential oil cream based on wild oils of oregano, lavender, and St. John's wort cures skin disorder

Ms. S. is a 35-year-old woman with a history of skin disorders, who works for a nutritional company. She had developed a dry, crusty patch on the side of her face, which seemed pre-cancerous. This made sense, as she was constantly exposed to the sun. She desired to avoid medical treatment and so tried a number of natural skin treatments, including Propolis Derma Cream and Yew Salve and similar medicaments made by her company. None of these were effective.

Within a few weeks, the lesion grew into a pea-sized lump, remaining crusty. The essential oil- and honey/propolis-based cream was applied. Said Ms. S., "The next day the crusty hard surface was softened, and the pea-sized lump was gone within another week." Thus, the natural cream consisting of raw honey, propolis, Canada balsam, wild oregano oil, wild lavender oil, wild myrtle oil, and wild St. John's wort oil, eradicated the lesion.

Relief of tennis elbow through oral intake of wild oregano oil

Mrs. J. suffered from a number of structural disorders, including pain in the knuckles and tennis elbow. She attributed these to strain from golfing and tennis. After reading about the powers of wild oregano in "The Cure is in the Cupboard" (same author) she took the oil of oregano, her dose only being three drops once or twice daily. Within 10 days, she reported, the tennis elbow syndrome was eliminated, while the knuckle pain improved significantly, about 90%.

Family stricken with Lyme disease-like symptoms cured with massive doses of wild oregano

Ms. H.'s entire family, her husband, herself, and her children—even her pets—were stricken with chronic infection diagnosed as Lyme disease. Ultimately, Ms. H.

became bedridden and was unable to perform even the most minimal tasks. She contacted me about a course of treatment. I recommended massive amounts of high strength oil of wild oregano, the essence/juice of oregano, the crude whole herb, plus natural flushing agents made from wild raw greens and wild raw berries. The dose of the oregano oil was enormous, some 40 drops three to five times daily. She was told it would take six months to regain her health. Incredibly, in six months she nearly fully regained her health, as did her husband and children. Now, she is able to function normally.

Oil of oregano under the tongue plus gelcaps reverse serious infection

Ms. D. is a 34-year-old with a history of cellulitis in her right leg. Antibiotics failed to reverse the condition. She began taking the oil of wild oregano, super-strong solution, along with the same strength in gelatin capsules. Within two days there was a noticeable improvement in the swelling and pain in the leg. Within a month the cellulitis was resolved.

Dire pain and infection reversed with oregano oil

Mrs. M. is a 75-year old woman with a previous history of debilitating shingles infection in her chest cage. Three years afterwards she awoke with shingles, this time on both sides of the chest cage. She did not think she could again face this dire pain. Fortunately, she had previously read the book the *Cure is in the Cupboard*. Following the advice in the book she took several doses of oil of wild oregano daily—and, incredibly, in two days she was "completely free" of the shingles.

Man with cardiovascular condition and diabetes undergoes radical improvement with crude wild oregano, red sour grape powder, natural crude food oils, multiple spice extract, and oil of oregano

Mr. J. is a 55-year-old male who is a stroke victim and also a diabetic. He was placed for several years on a number of medications, including a cholesterol-lowering drug, aspirin, and medication for lowering his blood pressure. After consultation, he began taking a number of natural supplements, including the oil of wild oregano, the whole crude herb, the red sour grape powder, the black seed oil, and the crude cold-pressed sesame oil (blue label brand). Within six months he was off all medication and then went to the doctor to have blood tests. The doctor reported that all the blood tests, including the blood sugar level, were normal.

Crude herb helps normalize a woman's bone structure

Ms. T. is a 65-year-old woman with a history of osteoporosis. She has tried the standard therapy for this condition to no avail. Reading about the high density of natural calcium and phosphorus in the whole raw oregano herb she began taking the wild oregano/rhus capsules, about six to seven per day. Prior to supplementation bone densitometry showed her bones as 25 years older than her age. After six months of wild oregano therapy using the calcium- and phosphorus-rich whole oregano herb she had another bone density test. This time she scored 25 years younger than her age.

Pink eye eliminated with spice oil spray

As reported by Ms. R. her 10-year-old boy had developed pink eye. Knowing the condition was likely caused by a virus she followed the advice I had given previously in my radio shows. She purchased the natural multiple spice spray, consisting of emulsified oils of oregano, bay leaf, and lavender and merely misted it over her son's head at some distance. This was to allow the mist to drift gently into the eye. Note: the solution should never be sprayed directly into the eyes but must be sprayed from a few feet away and allowed to drift downward into the face and eyes. Within 24 hours the pink eye was resolved. No other therapy was used.

Man kills tick with high (super) strength oil of wild oregano; aborts potential Lyme disease

Mr. K. is a 53-year-old male, who lives in southern Canada. While working outdoors he found ticks crawling on his clothes but removed them. Later that evening he felt something unusual behind his ear, where he found a tick attached. From reading the original book on wild oregano, the *Cure is in the Cupboard,* he knew the tick could be safely destroyed. Following the advice in the book he saturated a cotton ball with oil of super-strength oregano and applied it to the tick for several minutes, that is until it appeared obviously dead. Then, with a tweezers a friend pulled the tick from the tissues, and since the tick was dead, it was readily removed from the body.

Even so, the next day he developed a severe headache on the same side of the tick bite. This is likely indicates neurological involvement of the tick germs, where these germs invade the brain. As a result of the invasion of the brain and other organs Lyme or other tick-borne diseases could easily develop. Lyme is a highly serious condition which can lead to internal organ damage, including damage to the muscles of the heart. The brain is also readily attacked, particularly by the Lyme spirochete.

For Mr. K. there was a remarkable result. Frightened, incredibly, he took a half bottle of oil of wild oregano and held it in his mouth for several minutes. Then, he fell asleep. When he awoke, the severe head pain/headache was gone.

Combination of wild spice oils, including oils of wild bay leaf, and oregano plus cumin, fennel, and clove, eliminate digestive disorder

An Englishman, Mr. D., had a 20-year history of irritable bowel syndrome. He had tried virtually every known medical and non-medical treatment to no avail. He had taken numerous herbal medicines to resolve the condition to no avail. Believing it was parasitic he began taking a combination of the aforementioned spice oils in a base of crude cold-pressed pumpkinseed oil and extra virgin olive oil. Religiously, he took 40 drops twice daily. After 60 days of this therapy his irritable bowel syndrome was resolved.

Open wound on horse healed; side effect is improvement of crippling disease

In England a horse was crippled with laminitis, which essentially means the horse was lame. This horse, because of the crippling disease, was restricted by an enclosed space. Simultaneously, the horse developed an open festering wound on its cheek, which was being visited by flies. A super or high strength oil of oregano was squirted directly on the wound. Also, about 20 drops was squirted in the horse's mouth. What a noise the horse made when this occurred. Yet, he was fully cooperative. The treatment was repeated for three days. Rapidly, the wound healed. Plus, as a side effect the horse's lame condition improved dramatically, and after the third treatment he proudly pranced about to demonstrate his improvement.

Woman from Indiana has a curious side effect: while taking oil of wild oregano for a cold her other medical complaints are cleared

Ms. S. was plagued with chronic back pain for which medication was virtually useless. Having used oil of oregano successfully for colds in the past she had developed a sudden condition with pain in the throat and cold symptoms. She began using the oregano oil vigorously and after several days of treatment noticed that her back pain was eliminated. Note: oil of wild oregano, Mediterranean/aromatic-source, is a potent analgesic. It is also a powerful antioxidant and antiinflammatory agent. It is no surprise that it offers a diversity of positive effects on the body. With its analgesic properties it may be used as a topical rub but in Ms. S.'s case the analgesic powers were gained merely by oral dosing.

Aromatic multiple spice antiseptic spray offers unique benefit: acts as an ant repellent

Mr. L., a Californian, was having problems with an ant invasion. The invasion was sudden, and so he "grabbed the first thing in sight", which was a four-ounce bottle of the multiple spice spray. He sprayed the ants, and "they died instantly." However, he also sprayed around their colony site, and according to Mr. L., "They won't cross the barrier." Said Mr. L., "the results were amazing."

Severe psoriasis reversed; woman in tears

I was lecturing in Florida when a curious event happened. A woman in the second row began crying. Did I say something that offended her, I wondered? Then, after the lecture the woman immediately came up to me and began showing me the backs of her elbows and arms. They were clear with blotchy skin, where there was once severe psoriatic plaques. She then held up a bottle of a multiple spice complex made of dessicated wild and mountain-grown spices, oregano, cumin, and sage (also cinnamon), and said, "This is why I no longer have psoriasis." I diligently asked her exactly what occurred, and she said, again, that no other treatment had ever worked but this alone, this natural antiseptic spice concentrate, was responsible for her cure.

Teenager in coma awakened by wild oregano rub; potentially fatal septic shock averted

Mr. O. is a 17-year old, who was overcome by an infection by the notorious drug-resistant germ E. coli 0157:H7. This was contracted from contaminated water. The infection led to a condition known as septic shock, which is due to the toxic effects of bacterial poisons known as endotoxins. Also, the infection/toxin caused destruction of his red blood cells, which then caused both kidney failure and coma. There is no medical treatment for this condition. Without aggressive intervention through the use of a natural antidote the teenager would likely die.

His mother approached the doctors about the oil of wild oregano. The doctors refused to consider the use of oregano oil orally, despite the fact that the oil is proven to kill this germ. Thus, the teenager's mother decided to take action on her own by following my instructions and rubbing the oil in a high or super-strength version on her son's feet and chest. Within an hour the young man awoke from the coma and quickly said, "Mother, I think I can go home now." She continued the rubbing therapy and within 48 hours her son was discharged, the kidney failure and infection being completely resolved.

78-year-old man with pancreatic cancer experiences remission through oil of oregano

Mr. Y. was diagnosed with inoperable pancreatic cancer. His wife had heard about the oil of oregano through a radio program. She decided there was nothing to lose in trying it. Realizing the seriousness of her husband's dilemma she purchased the high (super) strength form of oil of wild oregano, along with the whole crude herb, in a capsule. She gave her husband 20 drops of this high strength oil twice daily, along with two capsules of the crude herb, twice daily.

Incredibly, within a week his pain and symptoms improved remarkably. Medical tests, she reported, ultimately showed him free of the cancer.

Man with poison ivy-like skin rash halts reaction with multiple spice spray

Mr. C. is a bushman who works in the far north of Canada. While in this environment he developed an itchy rash on his upper wrist. After scratching it he noticed the next day it had spread to his torso and upper forearm. He realized it was a reaction to a plant toxin and so began to spray the multiple spice oil on the lesions. He also rubbed oil of wild oregano on the involved regions (olive oil base). He did this repeatedly, up to 12 times in a day. Within the day the itching had nearly stopped and the rash stopped spreading. To speed the process up he applied saturated Telfa pads to the lesions, and kept them covered overnight. Within three days the rash had receded significantly.

Multiple wasp stings neutralized by oil of wild oregano plus multiple spice spray

Ms. K. is a woman who is familiar with the wilderness. She has regularly picked various wild berries from selected spots, but one year there was an 'epidemic' of underground wasp's nests, and she stepped on a nest and was severely and repeatedly stung. Immediately, she rubbed on the oil of wild oregano and noticed a significant reduction in pain. She kept using the oil and was able to neutralize the pain and inflammation within two days.

Symptoms of concussion eliminated with topical oregano

Mr. C. is a 53-year-old man, who struck his head on the edge of an overhead door. This caused a lump on his head and symptoms of a mild concussion, including dizziness, a feeling of unwellness, pressure in the nostrils/sinsuses, and a stiff neck. Nothing he took orally helped the symptoms. The neck stiffness was particularly severe. He reasoned that the wild oregano would solve this by halting the swelling. So he poured one-third of a bottle of super strength oil of wild oregano on his scalp over the lump and then covered it with a cap. Within a few hours the fogging of the brain, the neck stiffness and the dizziness had completely resided, as was the swelling of the scalp.

Blood clots dissolved with multiple spice extract

Mrs. K. was diagnosed with blood clots and, therefore, prescribed Coumadin. After unsuccessful results from the prescription drug, which gave her unwanted side effects, she quit the medication and instead tried two doses per day of the multiple spice extract containing extracts of cumin, sage, cinnamon, and oregano. After several weeks she reported that her blood clots were completely dissolved, and there was an additional 'side-effect', which was the elimination of the congestion in her chest as well as improved breathing.

Multiple spice extract reverses extreme allergy disorder

Ms. G. suffered for decades with chronic symptoms of allergy, including sore, swollen eyes, sneezing, and runny nose. In fact, while she wasn't aware of it these are also symptoms of fungal infestation. The runny nose and sneezing was virtually continuous.

The multiple spice extract as dessicated spice extract in capsules, was prescribed. As a result of the daily intake of these capsules she experienced "considerable relief" and had "such relief not to have to deal with the sore eyes, runny nose, and sneezing all day.

Nutritionist stung by a violent bee; welt and toxin eliminated with wild oil of oregano

While in a grocery store overseas Ms. G. was stung by an aggressive and large bee. This caused great stinging pain plus an immediate welt. She knew of the antivenom powers of oil of wild oregano and had a bottle in her purse. Immediately, she applied the oil and did so repeatedly. Virtually immediately the pain and swelling were decreased, and the stinging sensation was completely reversed. This was a dramatic result noticed by her husband, who observed a highly rapid reversal of this venomous sting.

Sales rep for major supplement company stricken with asthma; products from his company don't work; tries the multiple spice complex consisting of dessicated

with spice oil of oregano, sage, and cinnamon plus cumin. Asthma is eliminated.

Mr. N., an Irishman, is a 30-year veteran in the nutritional supplement business. Yet, despite being in the health field he was plagued with asthma, which is not an uncommon condition in Ireland with its high mold levels. On the health food store shelf he saw the label of the multiple spice extract with its prominent green label. So, he decided to try it.

His asthma was persistent and he was on a number of medications. Within 48 hours all his asthma symptoms were eliminated. Thus, he stopped all medications. Mr. N. was so impressed with the results that he proclaimed he was willing to change jobs and work for the makers of the multiple spice extract, the dessicated whole oil complex containing wild oregano and sage plus cumin and cinnamon. Said Mr. N. he had never had such a positive response to any other natural medicine previously. This, he said, was the finest natural product he had ever taken.

Husband and wife now cold and flu-free thanks to the oil of oregano

Mr. and Mrs. T. wrote me a letter praising the powers of oil of wild oregano. In the letter they said that they had suffered from generally poor health with various aches and pains and that they both had weak immune systems. Every year each of them would suffer from two or more bouts each of colds/flu. Since taking the wild oregano oil, however, there were dramatic improvements. They no longer caught every bug which came along and noticed that they, incredibly, had "more energy." Plus, there was the obvious and undeniable benefit of protection of the immune system, since they were no longer suffered colds and flu.

Consider this remarkable change. The couple knew this wild spice is a miracle medicine: from routinely getting sick with viruses every year to for over three years since beginning this natural medicine not getting even a sniffle. The oregano oil, they were sure, was the only reason for this change in their health. Mr. and Mrs. T. had tried a number of other natural treatments and said that no other natural medicine offered this exceptional power.

Woman with hepatitis C cured during clinical trial with high (super) strength oil of wild oregano

Ms. K. is an alcoholic, who developed hepatitis C. The cause of the infection was unknown, but the alcohol compromised her liver function. She entered a clinical trial using high (super) strength oil of wild oregano, along with wild raw triple greens extract. Within two years the liver function was normalized, and all traces of the virus were destroyed. The latter was proven by the measurement of normal, that is non-existent, hepatitis C viral titer, whereas before the oregano/wild greens therapy the viral titers were high at 5.5 million viruses per centimeter of blood. She received this cure despite the fact that she continued her alcohol habit, drinking against the doctors' advice several glasses of wine per week.

Man gets chest pain from noxious form of oil of oregano; uses the truly Mediterranean type to eliminate it

Mr. J. is a 50-year-old businessman who was at a health food trade show. Salespeople for a inferior brand of oil of wild oregano not based on research convinced him to try their product. This product, made by a Canadian company, caused Mr. J. to go into nervous shock with palpitations. He came to the booth for the original researched brand of oil of wild oregano (Mediterranean, hand-picked). There, he was given a few drops of the true oil of wild oregano under the tongue, which halted this reaction. Mr. J. then went to the booth of the inferior imitation type of oil of oregano and chastised them for putting on the market such an inferior (green-label) product.

Long-term colitis in 40-year-old man purged with wild oregano oil and whole crude herbal complex

Mr. K. is a physician with a history of colitis. This condition was related to stress but also a history of food poisoning when traveling overseas. No medication was of any aid in halting his disease.

A course of wild oregano oil plus the whole crushed herb with *Rhus coriaria* was initiated. He was instructed to take large doses of both supplements, the oil as drops under the tongue, about 20 drops three times daily plus the herbal complex as capsules orally, three capsules three times daily. Mr. K. noticed significant improvement within two weeks. Within two months the colitis was eliminated.

14-year-old female with undiagnosed TB almost killed by abdominal surgery; oregano saves her life

Ms. J. is a delicately built 14-year-old female, who developed a serious internal disorder. This was tuberculosis of the spine. A piano student she was being taught by a cancer victim, who had a lung disorder and may have contracted TB due to their close contact.

The TB manifested as an abscess along a muscle that is adjacent to the spinal column, known as the psoas muscle. This abscess caused such irritation that she was unable to walk and had to virtually crawl on the ground to move. The tuberculosis was housed in the vertebral column from which it formed fistulas (channels) and abscesses. Doctors noticed on scans the existence of abscesses along the spine/psoas muscle. So, they operated. This spread the infection and Ms. J. worsened. She was reduced to merely crawling slowly on the floor or ground to move. Despite this, both she and her mother were told by their surgeon that unless she had yet another operation to "drain the abscess" she would die. The mother wasn't convinced and so searched for answers.

After reading my book *Natural Cures for Killer Germs* the mother took action. She began giving her daughter massive amounts of oil of wild oregano (high or super-strength form), multiple spice extract, wild oregano essence or juice, a nine-strain special European healthy bacterial supplement, wild greens drops, and wild-source vitamin C. Gradually, there was improvement in her structural disorder due to the tubercular infection of the bones of the spine, and she was able to walk upright. However, she still was bent over to a degree due to the psoas inflammation. There are only two causes of psoas abscesses: one is fistulas in the intestines and the other is tuberculosis. In Ms. J.'s case it was clearly TB which was the culprit. After some six months of heavy wild oregano and multiple spice doses the abscess came to a head and an opening occurred, with fluids and toxins spilling from about the surgical site. This was the beginning of the prolonged healing process for this fine young girl, a process which surely saved her life.

Ms. J. is first in her class in academics. She is also a concert pianist. What a tremendous result for a young girl who under additional harsh medical care had little chance for survival. In intestinal and spinal tuberculosis surgery is contraindicated. Yet, the surgeons paid little heed to this and sought to continue invasive treatment. This would have virtually assuredly led to the death of this fine soul. All this was prevented by that high grade natural medicine, which according to the divine scriptures is a lifesaving substance.

Special note: for high dose therapy with wild oil of oregano: for all cases when taking large amounts of oregano oil and other spice oils there is a special consideration. Spice oils in large doses may kill the natural bacteria. Thus, when taking such doses over a prolonged period it is advisable to take a natural bacterial supplement on a regular basis. Also, it is advisable to consume extra amounts of yogurt, kefir, and quark or similar fermented milk products on a daily basis.

In Europe a particularly high grade healthy bacterial supplement is produced. This is known as the Ecologic 500 Probiotic Strain. This clinically tested group of healthy bacteria has an unusually high implantation capacity, which is ideal. Included in such a supplement are the following strains:

Bifidobacterium infantis
Bifidobacterium lactis
Bifidobacterium longum
Enteroccocus faecium
Lactobacillus acidophilus
Lactobacillus paracaei
Lactobacillus plantarum
Lactobacillus salivarius
Lactobacillus lactis

When using spice oils or other spice-based products this is the ideal natural bacterial supplement to consume. With antiseptic therapy using spice oils this is the ideal type of probiotic supplement to use. Search health food stores in the United States and Canada for such a supplement. Accept no inferior products. Also, this supplement is free of noxious additives such as genetically engineered vitamins, soy derivatives, and wheat derivatives. Ideally, such a supplement should be taken at a time away from the oregano or other spice extracts. The best time is at night at bedtime. This is only true when taking the spice oil concentrates such as the oil of wild oregano. It is perfectly acceptable to take the healthy bacterial supplement along with the whole crude herb, as found in the combination of wild crushed whole oregano leaf and *Rhus coriaria*.

These case histories demonstrate the diverse powers of oil of wild oregano and similar spice-based medicines. The use of spices as medicines dates to the beginning of human civilization. Even prior to civilization the spices were used medicinally. The first recorded use of spices as medicines is 50,000 years ago, as found in the tomb of an ancient princess. On the mummy's chest was found a sachet containing medicinal spices, primarily wild oregano. This was carbon dated at about 50,000-years-old. This is the oldest recorded use of spices as medicines. Since then all Mediterranean civilizations have used spices and their extracts as medicines.

Yet, the medical profession in all its glory has no understanding of this invaluable category of medicines. Simultaneously, hundreds of millions of people die needlessly every year from preventable diseases. There is no doubt about it because they lack the knowledge of the power of spice oils people die before their time. Even so, there is no possibility that modern medical authorities will back the wild oregano like, for instance, they backed the use of penicillin. This is despite the fact that research makes clear that regarding the saving of lives and the protection against life-threatening disease wild oregano extracts have far more potential than any antibiotic.

Chapter Four

A Healthy Environment

There is nothing healthier than pure air. In modern society this is a rare commodity. Many people spend the majority of their lives in highly polluted environments. Here, they breathe air which is unfit for human 'consumption.' As a result of the foul air respiratory conditions develop. Foul air also increases the risk of a host of other major diseases, including heart disease, joint disease, diabetes, and cancer. As a result of poor air quality the general health of people declines. Yet, there is a simple means to help rectify this situation. This is through the power of aromatic spice oils.

Spice oils are the aroma of paradise, so says the grand Qur'aan. This book also says that as a reward for good deeds there is a paradise, the breadth of which is more vast than the entire universe and its contents. In this paradise there is a drink, says the Qur'aan, with the a kind of gingery taste, which is exceedingly exotic and pleasant. In addition, it was the Prophet Muhammad who said that to keep the home purified essential oil-bearing plants should be burned, in particular, frankincense and wild thyme. In that era wild thyme was nothing more than wild oregano.

In the Old Testament wild oregano is mentioned as a cure-all, largely because of its ability to purge germs. This scripture urges people to use it for the treatment and prevention of disease. People are commanded, essentially, to "use" it. The ancient word for oregano is essop or ezov, which doesn't mean hyssop but, instead, means wild oregano. Again, this is known in the Middle East as wild thyme, which is also an erroneous distinction. So, what are people to do with the ezov? They are to "cleanse" or "purge." This is the purging of germs and toxins.

Historically, sprigs of this plant were placed in homes for purification. Church rituals today, where essential oils in the form of incense are burned, largely arose from their use for medical, not spiritual, purposes.

It is well known that essential oils help purify the air. This is critical, because the air can be poisonous. In the modern world it usually is toxic. This is particularly true of the air indoors. This is in homes but also workplaces. It is also true of the air in any other closed spaces, particularly airplanes, subways, and trains. In airplanes there is virtually no circulation of air. The same is true of many office buildings. Also, in many hotels there is no venting of air.

This is where decontamination is critical. In closed spaces there may be countless germs which can cause disease. There are also noxious gases which readily accumulate. In this air such germs and toxins must be neutralized. This can be achieved through the use of a wild oregano-based spray. Here, the powerful spice oils can be misted in an emulsified solution into the air to cleanse it. Testing at prominent institutions, such as Celsus Labs, proves that such emulsified spice oil sprays obliterate airborne germs, including mold, fungi, viruses, and bacteria. Such misting solutions, rich in phenolic compounds, offer another benefit. This is the decontamination of chemicals. Incredibly, the phenols are capable of actually neutralizing noxious substances in the air such as tobacco smoke, chlorine gas, cleaning chemical gases, airborne pesticide, diesel fumes, the gases from human breath, and car exhaust.

Again, a person can readily be poisoned by the air. This is because the air is the source of much disease. Think about a cold or the flu. Is not the air the main source of these diseases? What about tuberculosis? How can a person get this, without breathing? The same is true of sinusitis, pneumonia, bronchitis, asthma, and tonsillitis. Most of this is contracted from airborne germs.

Thus, every effort must be made to purify the air. This is an enormous protection against disease. It surely will help prevent sudden diseases, which cause so much misery and disruption. There is no reason to get colds, flu, sinus attacks, bronchitis, asthma, wheezing attacks, runny nose, and pneumonia. The wild spice oils in the form of sprays and as volatile oils will come to the rescue.

A multiple spice oil can be sprayed in any closed or unvented space to purify the air. Such a spray removes both germs and noxious chemicals. As well, volatile oils in an extra virgin olive oil base can be used, particularly in the home. Here, these oils may be carefully dripped into the melting portion of a candle; the flame of the candle will burn these off and the fumes will be invigorating. Of course, this is only true when using bees wax candles. Standard candles emit poisonous fumes, since they are made from petrochemical or coal tar derivatives. Also, be sure to only do this when the candles are secured, so there is no danger of causing fire, that is by accidentally tipping over the candle(s). Also, never leave candles burning unattended.

Another option is to add the oils to a diffuser. Too, there are special devices, which are available for burning such oils. The best oils for volatilization through burning are oils of wild oregano, bay leaf, lavender, and sage.

Another means of dispersing the oils is through using light bulbs. A device is available, a ring-like object, which can be placed over light bulbs. This is a brass ring with a trough. This trough can be filled with oil of wild oregano or similar spicy oils such as oil of wild bay leaf oil, oil of wild sage, and oil of wild lavender. One such device is called Home Essence Light Bulb Fragrance Ring and is made by Home Essence, Inc. of St. Louis Park, Minnesota, 1-800-516-6444.

Thus, a major effort must be made to cleanse the air of all impurities, particularly microbes. Dust is also a major cause of disease, as are noxious fumes. Both dust and chemical toxins damage lungs, while also suppressing the immune system in these organs. Infections can quickly develop as a result of exposure to foul air. By purifying the air the risk for the transmission of disease is greatly reduced.

Usually, fungi infect the surface tissues. This includes the skin and mucous membranes. Yet, in the extreme these organisms can attack all tissues. They easily infect the blood. Then, from here they can infect any tissue, including all the major organs. A major way to contract fungi is through the environment. Here, mold, a type of fungus, is found in the form of spores. The spores are inhaled, and once in the body they develop into their infective form. Another environmental fungus is the typical skin fungus from the family known as dermatophytes. "Derma" means skin. These are the organisms which cause toenail/fingernail fungal infections, jock itch, and athlete's foot. They are contracted via direct contact with surfaces such as the floors of showers, baths, and gyms.

Candida, the highly infective yeast, is also contracted through environmental contacts. In this case it is direct contact with humans, usually sexually. It is readily transmitted through sexual intercourse, but it may even be transmitted through kissing.

Airborne molds may also be transmitted through contact in tight spaces, where there is poor ventilation. A particularly high risk is airline air. Here, a person may inhale mold spores from an infected individual and, thus, develop a sinus or bronchial infection. Without some means of protection the risk for the development of a mold infection from such air is high. This is especially true if there are people on the airliner who have an active infection and who are coughing or sneezing.

In any closed region—airliner, home, public transportation, or office building—it may be presumed that the air is foul. The presumption is, thus, that this air could sicken a person. So, for prevention it is necessary to cleanse the air. This is through the methods which have been mentioned: the spice oil spray, the aromatizing ring, the candle technique, and, most importantly, the taking of the oil and the multiple spice complex orally. Fortunately, the spice oils eliminate all these toxic compounds. Regarding chemical fumes these oils, when volatilized in a spray, neutralize them. In particular, oils of wild oregano and bay leaf, as well as oils of wild lavender, cumin, and clove, in a spray emulsion neutralize tobacco smoke. These oils also bind and eliminate particulate matter, that is dust. Regarding the various airborne microbes tests show that the oils, when sprayed into the air, destroy these. In addition, burning the oils is effective in neutralizing noxious odors, although the burning process itself releases particles.

The spray, which is emulsified into a creamy liquid, can be regularly misted in the home as well as the workplace. The furnace filter can be misted. This should be done at least three times yearly and more often in homes which tend to accumulate dust.

There is significant insect repellent power of these oils. The misting of this emulsified spray on screen doors and screens in windows repels mosquitoes and other bugs. For picnics mist the air as needed with such a spray.

There is also a special spray specifically for repelling bugs. This is an herbal bug repellent, which is highly effective and highly aromatic. In a four-ounce bottle this contains emulsified oils of bay leaf, nutmeg, basil, lavender, and oregano.

Animal odors can also be reduced through these oils. Simply spray the area of concern, and repeat as often as necessary. Spray the under-belly of animals to control odors and to keep the animals from spreading disease.

Foul air is a major cause of sickness. Human odors are even more toxic than animal odors. With humans crammed into tight spaces, such as subways and airlines or even office buildings, disease can spread readily. This risk can be eliminated by the regular use of wild oregano-based sprays.

For burning in candles and light bulb rings the wild oil of oregano emulsified in extra virgin olive oil is the preferred type, followed by the oil of wild sage, oil of wild bay leaf, and oil of wild lavender, again in the base of extra virgin olive oil. Take such natural remedies with you whenever you travel for major protection.

Disease may also be transmitted through food and drink. Often, it is contaminated surfaces which are the issue. From these surfaces molds, bacteria, viruses, and parasites may be spread, leading to a wide range of illnesses, including diarrhea, flu-like syndromes, and inflammation of the liver. Or, the food itself may be contaminated. This is often through contaminated water. This happened in the United States recently, when so-called reclaimed sewage water was used in the farming of California spinach. The sewage water was contaminated with bacteria, a highly toxic form of E. coli, which were absorbed directly into spinach plants. In another similar crisis the stalks of green onions were contaminated by hepatitis B viruses; hundreds were sickened and several people died. This was also traced to contamination of the farming water. The viruses were lodged inside the plant, proving that water was the source of the poisoning.

Too, solid foods can be contaminated. Incredibly, salmonella infection has been contracted both through contaminated almonds and cereal.

Milk products may also be contaminated, especially cheese. This is particularly true of aged or strong-smelling cheese, which may be infected with Listeria. The same is true of luncheon meats, which may be infected with E. coli, staph, Listeria, or salmonella.

Commercial chicken is a common source of infection. The infection can develop both from eating the chicken and, perhaps, more commonly from handling it. Regarding the latter the chicken flesh or fluids may contaminate a surface and then other food is placed on that surface. If this food which is in contact with the contaminated surface is served raw, then, a serious infection may develop. Salmonella can cause fierce infections, and the germ may attack virtually any organ in the body, although the intestines, gallbladder, and joints often bear the brunt of the damage.

When preparing chicken, before baking, rub the carcass with a few drops of oil of wild oregano (Mediterranean, high-mountain source). Also, if making dressing or stuffing, add a capsule or two of the crude wild oregano with *Rhus coriaria*. After cutting the chicken spray and clean all cutting surfaces with the multiple spice emulsified spray. With such simple measures salmonella infection can be avoided. Even so, the best way to avoid it is to buy/consume only truly free-ranged chicken, which are never fed antibiotics, and it is this feeding of antibiotics in order to merely fatten farm animals which leads to mutated germs. Yet, even with this chicken since this bird is a scavenger, it is still a good idea to rub the carcass or its parts with a few drops of the oil or to sprinkle the parts with the wild crushed oregano/Rhus combination.

Thus, it becomes clear that food/beverage poisoning is no minor issue. In the United States alone some 95 million cases of such poisoning occur yearly. Attacks of diarrhea, stomachaches, liver pain/inflammation, and flu-like illnesses are all commonly caused by such poisoning. In fact, in the summer, when such attacks occur, food poisoning must be considered as the primary diagnosis.

Chapter Five

Children and Wild Oregano

It is a waste to allow a child to die prematurely. Yet, this happens to countless millions of children yearly throughout the world. Then, infection is the primary cause of such senseless deaths. Even so, virtually all such deaths are preventable. This is through the power of wild oregano and other spice substances.

Children love wild oregano. They know it is good for them. No child wants to take poisonous medicines. In this respect they are smarter than adults. Once they discover it they desire it. This is because, they know, it causes them to thrive. Plus, it preserves them, preventing them from developing painful or sudden illnesses.

A good safe whole food oil of wild oregano (Mediterranean hand-picked) can be safely used by children of all ages. This is true even of infants and toddlers. For newborns it can be safely used, either by rubbing it on the soles of the feet or by putting a single drop in a bottle of milk. Or, it may be taken by nursing mothers. Also, for any child eating solids the crude herb, combined with *Rhus coriaria*, can be added to boost both immunity and digestion.

Children learn quickly about anything that is useful. In other words they are self-protective. This is their natural condition. It is the instinct for survival.

How do children do this, when adults seemingly ignore the useful? It is because they are largely human interrogators. They seek to know why anything must be done. It is not enough to tell them anything; they always ask, "Why?" This is how they learn, that is to find the exact reason behind any issue. Here, they are often relentless.

To understand why any specific recommendation is important is how children learn. Adults should take note of this and realize the impact. In fact, adults, too, wish to understand the reasoning behind issues. Surely, this is true of medical treatment that could impact their very lives. Yet, children do it, instinctively. They automatically question the why. This demonstrates the natural tendency of the human to use reason.

It makes sense that if there are diseases on this earth that threaten human lives there are also cures. It also makes sense that the cure shouldn't be complicated and that, thus, anyone can apply it. Furthermore, it makes sense that such cures would be universal for all peoples and age groups and that while these cures are safe for adults, the majority are also safe for the tiniest of creatures, including newborns, infants, and toddlers.

Regardless, rather than any toxicity it is the consequences of not using natural cures, particularly oil of wild oregano, which must be of concern. Yearly, millions of children die prematurely from sudden infections. Through the powers of wild oregano virtually all such infections could be prevented. Surely, in prevention there are other factors as well such as sufficient nutritious food, safe water, and the intake of key vitamins such as vitamins C and A. Even so, in spite of deficiencies in these arenas the wild oregano will prove lifesaving. This is because it rapidly destroys virtually all germs, which cause sudden or life-threatening infections. The fact is wild oregano purges dangerous germs, and it does so quickly. Plus, it is broad-spectrum, meaning that rather than like antibiotics, which are isolated to a specific category, it kills all types of germs, including bacteria, fungi, parasites, and viruses. Thus, through this divinely-given medicine the sanctity of life can be preserved.

Again, compared to wild oregano, particularly the steam distilled oil emulsified in extra virgin olive oil, antibiotics are impotent. This is because antibiotics only kill certain categories of germs. Rather, in some cases they merely inhibit the growth of such germs. For instance, penicillin and its derivatives, such as ampicillin, only kill/inhibit bacteria. In children the germ which causes a given infection is rarely identified. Incredibly, in over 95% of all infections the actual germ(s) are never proven. So, in the majority of cases to contaminate infants, toddlers, and children with antibiotics merely because they have symptoms of infections is senseless. This is because in most cases there is no need for such drugs. What if the infection is caused by a virus? Obviously, the antibiotic will prove useless. Even more dire is if the infection is caused by a fungus. Then, the intake of the antibiotic will worsen the infection. This is never the case with the wild oregano. It cannot worsen any infection. Plus, whether the infection is caused by a virus, bacteria, or fungus is irrelevant. It kills all these germs. There is another reason the oregano is superior to antibiotics, which is the lack of side effects.

Children instinctively realize the power of wild oregano, but they also know it is safe. This is true only of the type derived from the whole mountain spice. This type is naturally pungent and spice-like, that is in its odor. So, toddlers and children, being instinctive, recognize that this is a natural and safe substance. In contrast, imitation types of oregano oil may have a bizarre odor similar to turpentine. Also, the taste is bitter or tinny. Thus, with these types the toddler or child might reject it.

With the true spice oil (Mediterranean hand-picked) there is no issue of danger. This safety is recognized by the children. It is only parents and doctors who fret about it. Consider little J., a two-year-old first born female child of a family in Iowa. Nearly dying from a vaccination, J. took a liking for the alternative, which is the edible spice extract oil of wild oregano (Mediterranean hand-picked). Whenever she had a potential infection before such an infection could gain hold her mother rubbed the oil on her feet and chest. This caused an immediate improvement, which the child noticed. She noticed that this substance was beneficial. Thus, now, she craves having it rubbed on her feet and chest, even when she is perfectly well. Yet, in the event she develops any symptoms of infection, she demands it, sitting quietly, as it is rubbed on her body.

Another story was related to me by a mother. Her children suffered continuously from bronchial and sinus infections. They also suffered from ringworm. All this means that the children had chronic fungal infection. Rather than the oil she gave them the crude whole herb by opening the capsules and mixing it with food. The sinus and bronchial infections disappeared, as did the ringworm. The children then began requesting the wild oregano regularly, especially if they felt ill. They love it so much they developed a nick-name for it, calling it "Maxie," standing for maximum strength wild oregano. This is the form of the whole herb, combined with the *Rhus coriaria*. Soon, the children also developed a liking for the oil, asking for it to be added to their juice. As a side effect they no longer develop colds or flu.

People may not realize it, but many antibiotics have serious side effects, including the potential for organ damage. In contrast, the spice-based oil of wild oregano is entirely safe for ingestion. All these comparative benefits are demonstrated in the following case history, in this instance involving a different tiny creature, a cat:

Antibiotic therapy causes feline diarrhea; cured by the crude whole wild oregano plus *Rhus coriaria*:

Mr. B. has a cat which he had treated with antibiotics for a cyst. This led to a significant case of diarrhea. The cat began losing weight due to fluid loss. Doctors only recommended additional antibiotics. I was consulted about this and told Mr. B. to halt all antibiotics and, instead, use the wild oregano. He added one or two capsules of the crude herb in the cat's soft food, which was consumed vigorously. After two oregano-enhanced meals the diarrhea stopped. Interestingly, after the condition was reversed the cat, which vigorously ate the oregano-food combination while ill, rejected any further treated food as soon as he was symptom-free.

Of all medicines wild oregano is, perhaps, the safest for children. It is safer than medicinal herbs such as goldenseal, echinacea, and horehound, even though compared to drugs such herbs are exceedingly safe. Oregano is a spice. Thus, it is a food. Just like curry powder it is, perhaps, more food than medicine. Think of it like ginger and cinnamon, that is as a food additive. This is even true of the oil and other concentrates such as the juice and multiple spice complex.

All are regarded by the body as food substances. Thus, these true foods are harmless to the internal organs. In contrast to drugs the wild oregano and other spice extracts are safe for the internal organs in the respect that they cannot cause organ failure. Rather, scientific studies conducted by one firm, which produces an extra virgin olive oil emulsion of Mediterranean oil of wild oregano, have determined that even in the event of liver disease wild oregano is not only safe but also curative. In the study conducted by A. Abdul Ghaney people with massive liver disease from hepatitis C were given large amounts of oil of wild oregano, up to 200 drops daily. In the majority of cases despite this enormous dose there was an improvement in liver function, as manifested by a decline in liver enzyme levels. Also, in most cases the levels in the blood of the hepatitis virus declined dramatically as a result of the wild oregano intake. Yet, the remarkable issue is that such a powerful substance caused in the majority of patients a normalization of liver enzyme levels. This means that not only is the oil non-toxic but that it also helps heal poisoned or damaged tissue. (Note: the type used in this study has the distinction of "Mediterranean wild, hand-picked in a blue and yellow label"— do not use any other for this purpose). Thus, it is an antidote, as is demonstrated by the following case history:

> Mr. M. is a 43-year-old male, who suffered from bronchitis. He heard about oil of wild oregano at a trade show and decided to try it. Rather than the original brand, which has been tested on humans and has undergone extensive animal testing, he took an imitation brand of questionable quality. Incredibly, his breathing worsened and he developed chest pain, sweating, and palpitations. Thus,

he experienced a toxic reaction. Then, this man came over to see me at a different booth, where I was signing books. Bravely, to reverse this toxicity I gave him five drops of the true oil of wild oregano from the wild Mediterranean spice. Within seconds, he dramatically improved. He then went to the other company's booth and chastised them for their inferior product.

This demonstrates the great value of oregano oil as an emergency medicine for children, as demonstrated by the following:

Ms. M.'s son has a serious dilemma, which is a peanut allergy. Whenever he ingests even a tiny amount of peanuts or other nuts he develops extreme welts. His lips swell, and he often develops throat swelling. She was instructed to give her child the wild oregano as the whole crude herb plus Rhus coriaria, along with the wild oil. As a result when her son accidentally ingests tiny amounts of nuts he no longer develops such symptoms.

Vaccinations or oregano: which is superior?

As mentioned previously children in particular take well to the wild oregano. They quickly develop a desire for it and a confidence in its abilities. Ultimately, as they experience it they want only oregano therapy, while rejecting all noxious medicines. Yet, regarding childhood illnesses do parents take such a natural approach with confidence? Often, parents "worry" and "fret" about what might happen to their children, often due to guilt. They feel compelled to, for instance, vaccinate, proclaiming, "If I don't and my child gets sick or dies, I will never be able to live with myself." This is not rational thinking.

What if the child gets sick from the vaccination? Do parents consider the dire risks, which are now documented? These risks include the development of type I diabetes, juvenile arthritis, anaphylactic shock, eczema, psoriasis, autism, attention deficit disorder, muscular dystrophy, mental retardation, pericarditis, paralysis, multiple sclerosis, Parkinson's-like diseases, leukemia, lymphoma, bone cancer, sarcoma, lung cancer, and brain cancer to name a few. Parents should consider, "Which is more threatening, the risk for such a chronic disabling disease or a mere case of measles, mumps, or pertussis?" Or, "Which is worse, taking the risk for the possibility of a virtually non-fatal communicable disease or developing a dire, essentially permanent condition such as leukemia, juvenile arthritis, type I diabetes, lymphoma, or brain cancer?"

Intuitively, the children realize this. Instead of shots and other invasive methods given the opportunity they crave the wild oregano. They will even ask for it, if getting sick. In contrast, they resist vaccination, and they also resist many medications. Here, too, they use their instincts. Consider the following child, who nearly died from a vaccination and her instinctive response to wild oregano therapy:

J., a rambunctious 2-year-old child from Iowa, had a wicked reaction to a set of vaccinations. Her mother was considering not vaccinating but due to fear decided to do so. At six months she received four vaccinations simultaneously and then developed wheezing, along with congestion. About a week later she suddenly stopped breathing, turning ashen gray, and was rushed to the hospital, fortunately being successfully resuscitated. Now, the parents are leery of vaccination and have halted them. Instead, they rely on the wild oregano, both the whole crude herb and the oil. If J. develops an illness, like an upper respiratory infection, she calls for the wild oregano oil. She asks for it to be rubbed on her feet. Rather, she demands for its use. Even when healthy she asks for the oil, saying "rub."

Why should children be vaccinated? Vaccines kill no germs. Moreover, there is no evidence that these injections prevent infections. To reiterate there is no proof of a preventive effect. Actually, rather than preventing any disease vaccinations create them. There are hundreds of diseases and syndromes which are directly caused by vaccinations. Furthermore, these injections are a major cause of sudden death as well as death from degenerative disease. Then, can a cure or preventive also kill? This makes no sense. If oregano killed people, would people be able to deem it a legitimate cure? If it killed even one person, could this spice be allowed on the market as a nutritional supplement? The answer is obvious, because, clearly, it would be banned. Yet, vaccinations are still systematically promoted as "required" despite the fact they routinely cause great disease and much death.

As mentioned previously vaccination is the primary cause of complaint to the government for sudden, serious illness. In a majority of cases SIDS (sudden infant death syndrome) is caused by vaccines. One death from these "trusted" injections is too many. Again, if a similar death in an infant, toddler, or child could be attributed to natural oil of wild oregano (from spice oregano) such a substance would be removed from the market. Yet, yearly vaccines cause thousands of deaths, and no action is taken? The corruption of the medical system is obvious for all to see.

Chapter Six

Finding the Right Oregano

The true wild oregano is a unique substance and is relatively rare. There are some 60 to 80 species of oregano-like plants. However, there are only a few species of such plants which are true medicinal forms of wild oregano. The true wild oregano grows in mountains on rocks or in rocky soil.

The sale of oregano oil began with a single product, which is of the highest grade. As medicinal oregano became popular this was diluted by inferior brands some of which are toxic. In contrast, the true wild oregano from the edible mountain-grown plants is completely safe for human consumption. This original product/supplement is derived from the wild oregano spice, which grows in the remote high mountains of the Mediterranean.

It is important to procure the original high quality spice as well as spice oil. Again, since the introduction of this highly regarded natural medicine there are on the market dozens of types of oregano oil supplements. Unlike the original type, as found in the blue and yellow label, none of such supplements have undergone scientific research. There have been no scientific studies done to assure safety. Nor has, unlike the original type, their effectiveness been studied.

Thus, taking any such supplements is a mere experiment at a minimum and may even prove dangerous, as demonstrated by the following case history:

> Mr. S. is a happy customer of the original form of wild Mediterranean oregano oil. After many months of using this oil and recommending it to friends he decided to save money by trying another brand. While surfing the net, he found a cheaper oregano oil claiming to be 100% pure. The oil claimed to be higher in the active ingredient than the famous type. He bought it, and gave it to his dog. Even though he diluted it 10:1 in olive oil the next day the dog died.

It is not just dogs who are sickened from untested and inferior supplements, as demonstrated by the following:

> Ms. T. is a woman of Romanian descent who is a big fan of natural medicine. This is all that she uses to treat disease and stay well. Now, living in Canada, she discovered oregano oil and found it effective for all infections.
>
> Her sister in Romania had fallen ill, so she decided to send her a bottle. However, the health food store was out of the nationally known brand, and so, instead, she purchased a 'competitive' brand (white label, as found in Canada) and sent it overseas. Her sister tried it, and fell into anaphylactic shock, nearly dying. After attending one of my lectures she asked how this could happen. I explained to her that there are corrupt forms of oils made from inedible plants or bizarre types of species, which no one eats. These plants are similar to wild oregano, but, again, no one eats them. Also, I informed her, there are

farm raised forms of wild oregano, and in this process
pesticides and herbicides are used. These noxious
chemicals are then concentrated in the distilled oil. I then
recommended that she send the true wild oil of oregano
made from the actual high mountain spice to her sister to
reverse the process.

I myself have experimented with such 'brands' to
understand what people are experiencing. One such brand is
promoted as being 100% certified organic and also wild. I
tasted it, and found it to be tinny in test, actually, highly bitter.
After taking only two drops I developed a severe pain in the
side of my head, followed by an violent headache. Also, I
developed a stomachache.

These symptoms were exceedingly severe. To eliminate
them I took the true oil of wild oregano under the tongue, five
drops every fifteen minutes. Within an hour all symptoms
were reversed. This was dramatic evidence of the power of a
true food-medicine versus an adulterated imitation.

When considering natural medicines how can a person
know the degree of quality? Surely, as one evidence the
company must truly care about the people. There must be
sufficient caring to avoid causing people harm. Any raw
material source, whether food or medicine, must be
carefully sourced to ensure quality. There must be every
effort to avoid the intake of noxious substances or additives.
What's more, there must be screening against contamination
by pollutants or toxic additives. This includes solvents, such
as benzene and hexane, which are used by some
manufacturers to extract the active ingredients. There is no
ultimate medicinal power in natural supplements made with
such noxious chemicals. The toxicity of the extracting

agent, mere derivatives of gasolene and kerosene, is surely greater than any medicinal power that can be derived from such an extract.

Consider dandelion leaves. These leaves contain a variety of natural substances, which exert beneficial actions on the body. In this leaf are diuretics, antiseptics, agents which purify blood, and also agents which stimulate the flow of bile. Ideally, the leaves are picked as spring greens and consumed, either fresh or properly preserved. When consumed, there would be a general benefit to the consumer. Yet, what if these leaves are treated harshly? What if they are cooked to high temperatures? More direly, what if they are soaked in noxious petrochemicals such as benzene and/or hexane? Would there truly be any medicinal action left—and true health-reviving powers—after such a treatment? Surely, the benefits would be minimal if any and would likely be overwhelmed by the harm.

With natural medicine quality first is the need. The natural medicines are made by the creator in a perfect state. In this state of perfection in which they are largely unaltered: this is where their true powers arise. When they are corrupted through violent treatment or the use of poisons, then, their powers are lost.

Again, consider the dandelion leaves. Anyone would like to eat fresh dandelion greens placed on salad. For the more adventurous these greens can be juiced for a kind of liver-gallbladder-purging tonic. Yet, would anyone eat such greens after they were soaked in benzene? Would anyone juice such greens as a beverage? Of course no one would do so. Yet, unwittingly, people are essentially doing this whenever they consume certain herbal extracts, particularly those made through standardization. Essentially, the chemicals used in producing such extracts "burn" the herb. For root or seed extracts the same harsh burning occurs. Regardless, a poison is surely unable to produce a medicine. Do not expect any powerful results from plant substances treated with chemicals, just as no curative results can be expected from foods contaminated with pesticides and herbicides.

Consider what happens in the wild with the animals. The wild beasts smell a given food. The same is true of any herbs, which they consume. If the food or herb has an off smell, they avoid it. In particular, deer are cautious of the food they eat, carefully scrutinizing their food sources. In a wild region an experiment in nature proves a point. The placement of commercially raised vegetables in a field grazed by deer found no takers, even though these vegetables were large and nutritious. Instead, the deer continued to graze on the native/wild grasses, while the vegetables rotted.

With oregano oil a number of corrupt practices may be maintained. The oil may be directly corrupted by the addition of sunflower oil and even kerosene. This is to extend it and keep the 'price' low. The finished oil may be whipped with a blender to force oxygen into it. This is to artificially raise carvacrol levels, the latter being an oxygenated phenol. Then, there is the issue of the refinement of the oregano oil. This is through a process known as fractional distillation. In this process certain components of the wild oregano oil are removed and sold mainly to the perfume industry. The rest, which is deodorized chemically, is sold as "essential oil of oregano." This is bought by various nutritional supplement companies and, then, converted into so-called Mediterranean oregano oil.

There is an even more dire issue. This is the labeling of oils as oregano oil, even though they are from completely unrelated species. There are some 80 different plants which produce oregano-like oils, including numerous species of thyme and marjoram. Commonly, the oils extracted from these plants are sold as Mediterranean oregano oil.

Finally, there is farm-raised oregano, which is usually various species of marjoram. These plants are raised either commercially or organically. Of course, the commercial type may be sprayed with pesticide and/or herbicide. The latter are concentrated in the distilled oil. Oils of marjoram are commonly labeled as oregano oil, and this isn't even illegal. Also, the name *Origanum compactum* is a species name for a type of marjoram, again farm-raised. Incredibly, *Origanum compactum* is not a true oregano species. Nor is *Origanum vulgare* the true oregano. Most oregano oils identified with the latter are, in fact, types of marjoram oils. The true oregano is a combination of various wild plants harvested by villagers in remote Mediterranean mountains. Rather than being identified by a species it is identifiable by the following:

- it is crude wild oregano, either as the crushed herb or as the extract—oil, juice, CO_2 extract, or dessicated spice oil
- it is guaranteed 100% wild spice oregano from the mountain chains of the deeper parts of the Mediterranean such as Turkey, Greece, and Syria
- it is notable by its rich robust smell and taste, which is never tinny
- carvacrol is not emphasized but, rather, the fact that it is a whole spice or extract
- again, that it is not identified in a generic way as *Origanum vulgare*
- that it is never identified as Mexican, Spanish, or Moroccan oregano

- that it is not hyped mainly for carvacol content instead of as a whole food supplement
- that it is never identified as a farm-raised version of wild oregano such as *Origanum vulgare.*

Note: Many farm-raised types, such as a number of imitation brands sold in Canada, are fallaciously labelled wild while, in fact, they are farm-raised.

There is another issue, which is rarely considered. This is the fact that in making a whole food oregano oil there is no one species, which is used. With the true wild oregano blend, which is sold as a premium brand in health food stores, wild material of a group of species and types is gathered from the mountain slopes. Thus, a true wild oregano oil is a blend of such species. Oils claiming to be made from a single species are usually farm-raised. Even more dire many of these are derived from genetically engineered types of oregano/marjoram plants such as those grown in Israel. Even so, unless it is truly wild material made from a blend of wild-growing oregano plants, then, the oil from such plants should not be consumed internally.

Now, unfortunately, genetically engineered variants of wild oregano are now commonly grown. An inquiry was made by the genetic manipulators or rather those who contaminate the genes to this author to assist them in their marketing. The offer was summarily rejected. These genetically engineered types are inherently corrupt and are, thus, unfit for human consumption. Unlike the true spice oregano there is no history of safety of use. The intake of such types is a mere experiment, whether the actual spice or the spice oil.

Again, the only type of oregano which is fit for human consumption is the truly wild material that grows naturally in the high mountains of the Mediterranean. This is a powerful yet delicate plant, which is sensitive to alterations in the ecosystem. It grows mainly on rock or the tiny bits of soil about rock. It doesn't easily grow on soil. What's more, it thrives particularly in the highest regions of the mountains, in fact, above the tree line. This is some 5,000 to 12,000 feet above sea level. Here, the oregano grows on the proper type of soil, which is essentially the by-products of white calcareous rock.

In other more outer regions of the Mediterranean the soil is entirely different. It is often reddish and is, therefore, completely different than the calcium- and phosphorus-rich soils upon which grows the true oregano. This true oregano will not grow in such soils/regions. Thus, beware of imitation brands, which are derived from non-oregano species—even though they are promoted as being true oregano. Instead, use only the original truly wild brand(s), which are guaranteed true oregano from the high mountain spice.

There are other reasons to beware when buying wild oregano. This is because of the introduction into the market of genetically altered species. These man-made versions of wild oregano are unsafe for human consumption. This is why it is important to only purchase the truly wild material, which is from regions of the Fertile Crescent. This is a certain means to avoid the intake of dangerous genetically engineered varieties as well as pesticide/herbicide-tainted farm raised varieties.

The true oregano comes from Lebanon, Greece, Syria, and Turkey. Regarding a source of the oil and whole herb these are the only reliable sources. In contrast, North African species as a source for the distilled oil are unfit for human consumption. So are those which are grown in North America. Beware of so-called oregano oil from Morocco, Spain, and Mexico. Again, these types of oregano are poisonous, as is demonstrated by the following case history:

> Mr. D. is a 50-year-old male, who is a big fan of oil of oregano. For convenience he shops at a local health food store, which produces its own brand of oil of oregano. Since it was labeled similar to the original brand, he thought it was of acceptable quality. After taking it he got an upset stomach, which occurred repeatedly whenever he consumed it. Also, he observed, it had a vile tinny taste, which was different than the previous type of oregano oil he had used. Upon further inspection of the label he noted that it said "made from Mexican oregano."

Yet, incredibly, there is no oregano naturally growing in Mexico, rather, only Mexican sage. The latter species, which is *Lippia gravolens*, is completely unrelated to wild oregano. Thus, it is fraudulent to represent this as an oregano plant. The oil from the Lippia plant has been associated with toxic reactions in a number of animals and, thus, should never be taken internally. This is a harsh oil and is from an inedible plant. Beware of this type of 'oregano oil.' Incredibly, it is falsely labeled and instead of being called oil of oregano it should be called oil of Lippia or oil of Mexican sage. For those who have purchased bottles and wish not to waste it there is a simple solution. It can be used in the household, for instance, as a toilet bowel cleaner or for cleaning mold from hard surfaces.

Why is such fraud occurring? There is, seemingly, a major market for wild oregano oil. This makes sense, since this potent spice is a natural antiseptic capable of killing all germs. Much of this movement was initiated by the original book on the subject, *The Cure is in the Cupboard* (Knowledge House Publishers, same author). Companies are attempting to capitalize upon this in every way conceivable.

Large nutritional supplement companies seek a standardized source. They do not regard genetic engineering as a drawback and seem, rather, to desire a type with standardized active ingredients. This is a violation of nature. In nature the plant produces a wide range of substances, never a single active ingredient. All such substances work together as a system, which accounts for the medicinal power and nutritional properties of the plant. This is proven by modern research. For instance, a study, published in *Molecular and Cellular Biochemistry* (Preuss and Ingram), was done in animals comparing the whole wild oregano oil (blue label material), the mountain grown type, compared to a synthetic version of carvacrol. The latter is a key active ingredient of the wild oregano. The animals were infected with yeast, and the oil of oregano and its synthetic version were given to prevent fatality, which they achieved. Even so, it was found that despite the power of concentrated carvacrol the whole distilled oil was twice as effective. Yet, there was an additional finding. This was the fact that the whole spice oil is non-toxic, while the synthetic concentrate had a degree of toxicity. This again proves that whole foods and their extracts are entirely safe for human consumption and that, in fact, it is unsafe not to make use of them.

The true spice and its derivatives, including the highly potent steam distilled oil, are entirely safe for human consumption. Plus, such pure, natural foods/extracts can be consumed with impunity, that is they can be consumed in large amounts, as needed. Consider the safety of a true spice-based oil of wild oregano. Blood tests of numerous humans who have taken relatively large amounts, for instance, 40 or more drops daily, prove an astonishing finding. Rather than any toxicity there is, in fact, dramatic improvement in blood chemistry. In a number of instances the blood chemistry profile was exceptional.

Rather than such a whole pure substance it is the noxious germs which must be feared due to their toxicity. The wild oregano, the true spice mentioned in ancient scripture, is, perhaps, the safest natural medicine known. In fact, rather than merely safe it is lifesaving. In the Bible it is mentioned as a purging herb, obviously referring to its potent germicidal property. It is likely that this scripture refers to the antifungal powers of wild oregano, since fungus is a primary contaminant of the human body. To purge fungal organisms from the human body is a true boon, resulting in massive improvements in health. Scripture knew what modern science remained ignorant of, that is until recently, which is that billions of humans suffer from chronic mold infections in their bodies. These molds are not easily eradicated, therefore demonstrating the need for a purge.

The Qur'aan, too, mentions spices, deeming them purifying agents. This is because this scripture says that the beverages of paradise are purified or flavored with spice, as is the air. As mentioned previously the essence of one of the drinks of paradise is described as exotic and ginger-like, with a flavor unknown to humans. Here, clearly, spices, with their profound aroma and taste—and with their ability to purify all corruption—are regarded as godly.

It is now known, as a result of studies done at Celsus Labs, that this is precisely the case—that spice oils misted into the air destroy all traces of germs, particularly those responsible for the creation of noxious fumes. Regarding the Bible's claim of oregano as the purging herb this is also confirmed by scientific investigations. It was again work performed at Georgetown University, published in *Molecular and Cellular Biochemistry*, which demonstrated this, when the oregano oil was proven to purge all traces of a highly infective fungus, the human strain of *Candida albicans*. It only took 30 days to purge all traces of this yeast from the tissue. No other natural substance was found to achieve this. Thus, the wild oregano stands alone as the agent of power for purging various noxious forms of fungi and mold, which infect the human body.

These scriptural statements are fascinating. In particular, they must cause scientists, who might deny the existence of the higher power, the One who creates the universes, reservation. How could people in ancient times know these facts? This proves that this universe is created with a purpose. One such purpose is to provide the human being with all his needs, including the various natural medicines which can cure disease. Obviously, the God of this universe cares much for His creation and actually wants people of this world to be well. This is because He is truly the most merciful Being conceivable. Whoever wishes to believe in this may believe in it, and whoever wishes to refuse it will refuse it.

Even so, why else would He mention exactly what they need to do to regain their health? This is to take spice oils to obliterate all traces of infection, including those infections which are the cause of chronic disease. This is through the intake primarily of wild oil of oregano, the crude whole oregano spice, and possibly the essence or juice of oregano.

It is also through the intake of other similar spices, which are, incidentally, also mentioned in scripture, including cumin, black seed, and possibly sage.

Regardless, all such spices were used by the ancients for powerful health and also to prevent aging. Modern humans should take advantage of these so they, too, can be in superb health. It is also so that they can gain the power they need to avoid succumbing to dire consequences. These are the consequences of premature death from preventable diseases such as pneumonia, fungal infections, blood poisoning, dysentery, asthma, flu, encephalitis, meningitis, tropical diseases, and bacterial infections. All such potentially fatal infections are both preventable and curable with oil of wild oregano.

For prevention the oil can be taken daily. Even small amounts, like two drops under the tongue or in juice/water, are preventive. Ideally, the whole crude herb in a capsule should be taken, along with the oil. Here, it must be remembered that microbes readily attack the human body and these microbes may do so chronically, that is they may fail to elicit an immune response. So, this daily intake of the wild oregano is not merely to prevent colds, flu, and sore throat. It is also to prevent the development of chronic disease.

In fact, there is a significant connection of infection to chronic disease. So, the regular intake of the wild oregano is an insurance plan against such diseases. A list of diseases associated with infection includes arthritis, lupus, scleroderma, psoriasis, eczema, seborrhea, diabetes, rosacea, heart disease, mitral valve prolapse, cancer, vasculitis, nephritis, gastritis, colitis, thyroiditis, and pancreatitis. Even certain neurological diseases are tied to infection such as multiple sclerosis, Parkinson's disease, ALS, and Alzheimer's disease. As well, schizophrenia and manic-depressive syndrome may have an infection connection. The same is true of autism and attention deficit syndrome.

There is a major reason this must be emphasized. It is because most people don't consider infection regarding such conditions. Thus, the treatment rarely if ever includes substances for purging germs. Ideal substances for such purging include the oil of wild oregano, the whole crude herb/spice, oil of wild/edible sage in an extra virgin olive oil base, and the watery essence or juice of oregano. For neurological diseases the purging of germs may prove lifesaving, as is demonstrated by the following case history:

> Mr. H. is a 60-year-old man who was completely incapacitated. Diagnosed with ALS or Lou Gehrig's disease, he was paralyzed and wheel-chair bound. Mr. H. was unable to move his arms or legs.
>
> By the good graces of his neighbor he was given a bottle of wild oregano juice (steam extract). Incredibly, after taking a mere tablespoon within an hour he was able to move his right arm. An hour later he was able to move his left arm. Within three hours he was able to stand up and walk. Then, he walked together with his wife to the kitchen, where they cried together and hugged each other. He is now able to work full time on odd jobs about the home. In fact, his agility returned to such a degree that he was able to repair the roof on his house. This is a spectacular result for such a simple therapy. The cure was entirely the oregano juice, which was taken in the modest dose of a tablespoon daily.

Germs readily infect all organs, including critical structures such as the brain, spinal cord, kidneys, and heart.

Incredibly, no organ is exempt from such infections. On autopsy it has been found that virtually any organ may be infested with germs, much of this occurring, without obvious symptoms. Surely, these infections contributed to premature death, but no one realized it.

In postmortem examinations even worms have been discovered in key organs, such as the heart and liver, without obvious symptoms. Also, it has been found that even the hormone glands, the thyroid, pituitary, and adrenal glands, can be chronically infected to the degree that the infection is only discovered upon autopsy. This demonstrates the immense value of the use of natural antiseptics, such as oil of wild oregano and multiple spice complex, in the prevention and reversal of disease. The infections are inherently established within the body. There are often few if any symptoms. The person may merely be tired. There could be swelling and bloating. There could merely be abnormalities in blood tests such as high cholesterol, C-reactive protein, sedimentation rate, or white blood cell count. There could also be vague pain, like joint aches and stiffness of the back or spine. There could also be skin disorders. In most instances all this is eliminated through the intake of wild oil. Thus, the natural antiseptics may be taken routinely for creating good health as well as maintaining it. This may explain the true meaning of the scriptural command to "purge."

No doubt, purging hidden germs from the body will boost health. These are stealth invaders which cause great damage to the immune system as well as the internal organs. Such germs include fungi, molds, mycoplasma, cell wall deficient bacteria, staph, strep, amebas, worms, and protozoans. Once the germs are neutralized, the functions of the body will be more balanced. There will be an increase in energy. The desire for exercise will increase. The germs drain great energy from the body. Once they are killed the energy and vitality returns. Fatigue is essentially eliminated. Through the destruction of such pathogens inflammation is also eased. So is joint swelling and deformity. The complete destruction of invasive organisms may even result in a normalization of the joints, both in appearance and function. While it is little realized, gross deformity of the joint, as seen in arthritis and, particularly, rheumatoid arthritis is largely due to persistent infection. The culprit is usually parasites, which infest the gut and liver, ultimately damaging and even invading the joints. However, fungi can also cause this. This is particularly true of swollen and/or deformed knuckles, which is virtually always a sign of intestinal infection, again, by either fungi or parasites. Stiffening of the hands can also be due to internal infection.

Chapter Seven

The Fungal Epidemic

There is no doubt about it fungal infection is a massive cause of human disease. It is completely abnormal to have fungi in or on the human body. It is a sign of toxicity and, therefore, weakened immunity. Fungi are vile germs which thoroughly poison the body. These organisms should never be in the blood or internal organs. They should, ideally, never be growing on the skin, hair, scalp, or nails. That is true evidence of a sickness.

Fungi produce a vast number of poisons. They actually secrete these poisons into the blood and other tissues of their hosts. These poisons neutralize the host's immune system. They sicken people. The poisons interfere with the function of virtually all organs of the body. Even so, in particular the fungal toxins cause the immune system of the host to become incompetent. This is so the fungi can gain a foothold and so they can, then, permanently infect the body. These organisms are parasites, and like all other parasites they seek to take control of their hosts. When they do so in humans, they drain enormous amounts of energy from the body, and this leads to disability and disease. Thus, conditions, such as chronic fatigue syndrome and fibromyalgia, are often caused by fungal infestation.

There are people who have countless trillions of fungal organisms living in their bodies. These people are truly sickened, and the only way for them to regain their health is to decimate these levels of fungi. This is by taking the oil of wild oregano, as well as the multiple spice extract, on a regular basis. It is also by taking a high quality probiotic supplement. Then, they will systematically purge all traces of the fungi from their bodies, although it may take a prolonged time.

There are other oils, which can be added to the protocol for fungal purging. These oils include oil of wild myrtle, oil of cumin, oil of wild sage, and oil of wild bay leaf. This may be found as individual oils in an extra virgin olive oil emulsion, ideally as edible spice oils. For additional purging power these may be taken, along with the oil of wild oregano, as drops under the tongue.

How is it known that there is an epidemic of fungal infections? Again, it is the modern lifestyle, which is largely responsible. The food that is consumed is the culprit, along with indoor living, lack of sunshine, the overuse of antibiotics, the excessive intake of cortisone, plus excessive stress. All these cause or aggravate fungal infection. There are countless billions of people who are sugar addicts. Thus, there are countless billions of people who have fungal infections. The same is true of the billions who regularly take antibiotics.

The warming of the planet has also contributed to the increased incidence of this infection. Fungi/molds thrive in warm climates and love moisture, while cold tends to destroy them. Flooding of buildings, of course, leads to mold growth, which may cause devastation of health. There are a number of highly toxic molds, which grow in water-damaged buildings. Moreover, these molds may be hidden, as the mold grows readily in dark or inaccessible places. Then, the constant exposure to mold toxins or, in fact, the actual inhalation of the molds leads to disease. Diseases/symptoms that may be caused by hidden—or obvious—mold infestations include asthma, wheezing, bronchitis, sinusitis, pneumonia, headache, spinal stiffness, joint aches/arthritis, skin disorders, chest pain, nose bleeds, depression, anxiety, hallucinations, seizures, and psychosis.

There are also the diseases, which are clearly due to fungal infestation. Many of these diseases have already been mentioned. Certain of these diseases have been definitively proven to be caused by fungi and not by, as has been commonly believed, bacteria or viruses. These diseases of virtually definite fungal origin include sinusitis, bronchitis, allergic rhinitis, chronic serous otitis media, Sjogren's syndrome, psoriasis, eczema, diabetes, fibromyalgia, chronic fatigue syndrome, autism, chemical sensitivity syndrome, and asthma. Categorically, these are fungal disorders, although there may be secondary factors such as chemical toxicity and/or food intolerance.

In creating the vulnerability to fungal infection toxic overload of the body may play a significant role. This is because this toxicity, then, feeds fungal overgrowth. Too, there are the conditions which are obviously caused by fungal infection, including toenail and fingernail fungal infestations, ringworm, jock itch, and athlete's foot. As mentioned previously vitiligo and alopecia have now been proven to be fungal in origin. Stress is also a significant factor, since this depresses immunity, creating the potential for fungal overgrowth.

Obviously, in a truly healthy person it would be difficult for fungal organisms to infect the tissues. Yet, where on this earth is there a truly healthy person? There is such a great deal of stress affecting people plus toxic diet. Even if the diet is not completely toxic, still, there is plenty of reason for fungal overgrowth. This is because the majority of people eat an excess of carbohydrates. This is far in excess of the amount eaten by ancestors or even the amount the body can handle. The excess carbohydrate is converted to sugar, which feeds fungi. Moreover, the majority of people consume massive quantities of sugar, not just as refined sugar but also in many other forms such as malt syrup, maple syrup, honey, rice syrup, corn syrup, and fructose. All this sugar feeds the growth of fungi within the body. So, there is plenty of reason to go on a fungal purge—for virtually all people, with very few exceptions.

The purging of fungi is assisted by cleansing therapies. The reduction of poisons in the body enhances the fungal kill, since these parasites thrive on filth. The ideal types of cleansing methods include, possibly, enemas and foot baths. Bentonite clay may also prove therapeutic. Regarding foot baths it is the ionic type—the electrical foot baths now commonly being used—which are most useful. The pores of the body are largest on the bottom of the feet, and this is useful in the purging of toxins.

Perhaps even more powerful is a direct purge using wild raw greens extracts plus heavy monounsaturated fats. This is a potent way to eliminate poisonous matter. Remember it is such matter, lodged within the body, that facilitates fungal growth. Most of this morbid matter is lodged within the liver and spleen as well as to a degree the kidneys. Thus, the ideal purge focuses on cleansing these organs. Such a purging agent is available as a 12-ounce bottle containing wild raw greens extracts, wild high cranberry extract, black seed oil, extra virgin olive oil, raw apple cider vinegar, and spice oils.

There is also a wild raw greens flushing agent that can be taken as drops under the tongue, consisting of extracts of wild nettles, dandelion leaf, and burdock leaf. These drops are raw.

Black seed oil is highly cleansing. The regular intake leads to an increase in the production of bile. It is the bile that is the body's natural soap, which acts to cleanse the intestinal wall. Bile is also a natural germicide. Furthermore, it is necessary for normal fat digestion. People who are intolerant to fatty foods usually produce an insufficient amount of bile. As well, extra virgin olive oil provokes bile production, yet black seed oil is more potent in this regard. The wild bitter greens—the nettles, dandelion, burdock, chickweed, clintonia, and fireweed—all stimulate bile synthesis. So do certain spice oils such as oils of fennel, sage, rosemary, and coriander.

Bile is the body's means for the detoxification of dangerous chemicals. A vigorous increase in bile leads to the elimination of poisons from the body. In addition, bile helps the body mobilize heavy metals such as mercury and lead. Thus, boosting bile synthesis is an ideal and safe means to purge such dangerous metals.

The purging of such metals can prove lifesaving, as is demonstrated by the following case history:

Mrs. J. has a 10-year-old son who is severely autistic. The child was unable to function normally in any respect, including interacting in school. She reasoned that he was poisoned by vaccinations, both by vaccine viruses and also mercury. She began a treatment protocol of wild oil of oregano and a triple greens flushing agent, which is well tolerated by children as drops in juice or under the tongue. Within four days there was a dramatic result: the child passed a massive stool, which was dark green in color. This apparently liberated much of the child's toxic load. Subsequently, that day the child requested exercise; he did forty minutes on a treadmill. In school for the first time he participated in recess, playing for over an hour, well over the allotted time.

It should be no surprise that such natural substances are effective, as well as safe, for children. The powers of extracts of nettles and dandelion, as well as wild oregano, have been respected for centuries. Regardless, rather than actual medicines these are whole foods. Grieve in her classic *A Modern Herbal* describes nettles as in general stimulating body functions as well as assisting in tissue regeneration. Dandelion, she notes, is highly specific for kidney and liver disorders. It is even effective, that is the root extract, for purging gallstones. Even for certain infections, including fungal infections and the fungus-like tuberculosis infections, dandelion, as well as nettle, says Grieve, has proven effective.

This emphasizes the benefit of combining the wild spice oil therapy with the purging/cleansing therapy based upon wild raw greens extracts. For information on such extracts see Americanwildfoods.com. Available at this Website are the raw wild greens drops, wild nettles extract, wild dandelion extract, and wild fireweed extract. There is also a super-five greens beverage available for drinking as a morning raw greens beverage (about an ounce or two in juice or water). Thus, there are, now, a wide range of raw wild greens foods available. It is the greens in the raw state that act as natural antifungal agents as well as powerful cleansing agents. Both raw wild dandelion leaf and raw wild nettle leaf contain antiseptics such as formic acid and saponins. For instance, the milky cream that oozes from a broken dandelion leaf is an antiseptic. Even so, the basic protocol for purging fungal infection from the tissues is as follows, this being the "basic" protocol:

- oil of wild oregano, high (super) strength: 10 or more drops three times daily
- multiple spice complex, consisting of dessicated oils of wild oregano, sage, cumin, and cinnamon: one or two capsules three times daily with meals
- the crude whole wild oregano herb, along with *Rhus coriaria*: two or more capsules three times daily
- the watery extract (steam-extract) of wild oregano (for those with neurological symptoms): a half ounce daily
- a potent purging agent consisting of raw wild greens in a base of black seed oil and extra virgin olive oil plus aromatic spice oils: an ounce or more daily before breakfast (note: this purge should be continued for at least 24 days)
- a wild raw triple greens flushing agent, as drops under the tongue: 20 drops twice daily
- a wild raw lingonberry extract, which is especially of value for fungal infestation of the heart, kidney, bladder, and prostate. It can also be used vaginally.

In addition, when taking such high doses of oil of wild oregano a healthy bacterial supplement should be consumed. This should be taken at night before bedtime. Other food supplements which would prove helpful in the eradication of the fungal infestation include oil of wild myrtle, oil of cumin, oil of sage, and oil of bay leaf. Many such oils are found in the aforementioned multiple spice complex. Even so, these oils may be purchased as extra virgin olive oil emulsions for use sublingually. As well, extracts of wild nettles, dandelion leaf, dandelion root, and fireweed are all to a degree antifungal.

Wild raw berries extracts, such as a multiple raw wild berry extract, as well as single wild berry extracts, also exhibit antifungal properties. The wild raw berries extracts, again, as drops under the tongue, offer the additional benefit of regeneration of the circulatory system. Thus, these berries extracts help boost blood flow. This causes an increase in oxygen to the tissues, which greatly assists in the destruction of deep seated fungal infections. Also, toxins are cleansed, allowing the tissues to be revived. Wild berries with particularly potent antifungal actions include wild raw high bush cranberry (honeysuckle) extract, wild raw chokecherry extract, and wild raw black raspberry extract. In addition, wild raw currants possess antifungal properties. Other antifungal wild berries/fruit include wild camu camu and wild palm fruit. The latter are found in a high grade supplement made from wild Amazonian fruit, including wild raw camu camu, again, as drops under the tongue.

Oils are antifungal. Also, in contrast to high sugar fruit and starches oils and fats never feed fungus. Thus, fatty foods and various supplemental oils are ideal for the antifungal diet. Also, essential fatty acids in particular are antifungal. These are the fatty acids and linolenic acid. Excellent sources of such fatty acids include primrose oil, black currant oil, pumpkinseed oil, walnut oil, flax oil, wild sockeye salmon oil, and the highly potent Amazonian sacha inchi oil.

The antifungal diet

The antifungal diet must be low in sugar and starch. Correspondingly, it must be high in fat and oils. It must also be high in protein. The protein helps elicit stomach acid, which is highly antifungal. Without stomach acid the fungi/yeast in the food cannot be killed. Such a diet helps starve the fungi. Sugars must be limited to the natural sugars/starches found in vegetables and certain fruit. The fruit must be low in sugar. The antifungal diet should be followed strictly for 90 days. The following foods are ideal on such a diet:

- organic or grass-fed beef, bison, elk, and venison
- organic poultry, particularly turkey, goose, and duck
- fish of all types
- seafood of all types
- organic eggs
- organic whole milk products, particularly yogurt, heavy cream, cottage cheese, and farmer's cheese (avoid all fermented cheese)
- dark green vegetables
- tomatoes
- avocados
- sour fruit (lemons, limes, grapefruit)
- berries (strawberries, blueberries, black raspberries, cranberries)
- pecans, macadamia nuts, pumpkinseeds, walnuts, filberts

Note: Yacon syrup and stevia are the only sweeteners allowed on this plan. The only juices which are acceptable are tomato, V-8, raw greens juice, Super-5-Greens Juice (raw and wild), and, perhaps, pure unsweetened cranberry, lemon, lime, and grapefruit juice). Regarding yacon syrup be sure to buy only the truly raw unprocessed type, Peruvian-source.

Wild nut extracts are another key component to this diet. Wild nuts are rich in tannic acid, and this is especially true of the shells. Extracts made from a combination of the nut and shell, are not only nourishing but highly antifungal. Such extracts can be found on Americanwildfoods.com. These extracts are made from wild hazelnuts and hickory nuts. The nourishment value of these extracts is exceedingly high, since they contain a dense amount of trace minerals, notably calcium, magnesium, and potassium, as well as large amounts of highly nourishing monounsaturated oils and vitamin E. The vitamin E is largely found as gamma tocopherol, which is the most potent form in terms of antioxidant powers.

So, a person can follow this diet, along with the wild oregano and spice oils as well as the natural purging agents. For additional power the wild berry extracts may be taken. This is sufficient to ultimately reverse all fungal disorders. Even so, it is important to realize that this may take time. It may take as much as six months to destroy the fungus. Thus, persistence is necessary. Eventually, the cure will be achieved. Also, in extreme cases it may be necessary to increase the dose, perhaps, doubling or tripling it. This is true of all the supplements, including the purging greens, the berries, and particularly the spice oils. There may also be a need to add additional antifungal oils such as oil of wild myrtle, oil of wild bay leaf, and oil of cumin. Here, as much as twenty drops of each twice daily can be taken to accelerate the destruction of the pathogens. As well, many of these oils are found in dessicated form in the multiple spice extract, which is particularly ideal for respiratory disorders caused by fungi such as asthma, bronchitis, and sinusitis. Remember, these are highly invasive germs, which are deeply infective. Thus, a most aggressive approach must be taken to achieve a true cure.

Basic diet for oregano therapy

The diet for people taking the oregano should be relatively high in fat. The wild oregano operates best in a fatty medium. The fat assists in the absorption of the oregano active ingredients through the lymphatics. So, the oregano's oil works best, as does the crude herb, when taken with a fatty meal. A low fat diet is the poorest type to consume when doing oregano therapy.

In contrast, organic butter, whole fat milk, yogurt, free-range eggs, poultry, and red meat are ideal foods for oregano therapy. Again, the fat is needed for the absorption of the active ingredients, the essential oils, of this spice. Because of their rich content of antioxidants vegetables and fruit are also ideal foods on this plan. They also work synergistically with the oregano, as do the wild berries extracts. Supplements which help potentiate the power of the wild oregano include:

- a wild triple greens complex containing extracts of wild burdock, nettles, and dandelion
- essence of wild nettles
- a purging agent based upon oils of black seed and extra virgin olive oil, along with extracts of wild greens, wild high bush cranberry, and spice oils
- a wild raw eight berries extract consisting of various

wild raw berry concentrates, including wild black raspberry, wild red raspberry, wild chokecherry, wild blueberry, and wild service berry (saskatoon berry) extracts
- fatty medicinal oils such as crude cold-pressed sesame oil, black seed oil, and extra virgin olive oil
- separate wild berries extracts (cold-processed) such as extract of chokecherry, blackberry (or brambleberry), black raspberry, red raspberry, lingonberry, and wild/high bush cranberry.

Toenail fungus: the latest research

This is not just a cosmetic issue. Toenail, as well as fingernail, fungus is a sign of systematic disease. This is a disease of the immune system and, therefore, fungal overload. It is toxic, and for ideal health the condition must be resolved.

Spice oils are the treatment of choice for this condition. This is because these oils are safe for internal consumption—long-term consumption—which is required to eradicate this chronic condition. Plus, they offer the ability of topical use. Furthermore, they are the most potent antifungal agents known.

There is good science to confirm this. Toenail/fingernail fungus is caused by a group of fungi known as dermatophytes. In this regard a powerful study was conducted at Georgetown University. The pathogens which cause toenail fungus were put in the petri dish. Natural treatments, as well as drugs, were tested. The drugs were griseofulvin, fluconazole, and terbinafine (Lamisil). The natural medicines were oregano oil, clove oil, cinnamon oil, and bay leaf oil, along with monolaurin. It was determined that oregano oil and bay leaf oil were four times more effective in killing the fungus than most of the drugs. Lamisil was slightly more powerful than a blended oregano oil, but when a combination of the natural spice oils was used, it proved more effective than the drug. Lamisil, while potent, has significant side effects, including permanent liver damage. There are no such side effects with the spice oil combination. This spice oil combination is available in a one-ounce dropper bottle in a base of extra virgin olive oil and sacha inchi oil, as well as in 240 mg gelatin capsules (blue label brand). A human trial is currently being conducted, which will likely show similar results.

Chapter Eight

The Science

There is a great deal of science supporting the power of wild spice oils. This science includes a significant amount of human research. Yet, the greatest science is in human use. Spices and their extracts have been used as natural medicines from the beginning of human existence. Regarding organized societies there is major evidence of use, for instance, in 5000 to 3000 B.C. by the Sumerians and Babylonians. Here, in particular wild oregano was used for infections as well as heart disorders. The ancient Greeks relied on wild oregano for all wounds as well as venomous bites. For internal disorders they found that this wondrous natural medicine, which they named *oro ganos*, which means delight of the mountains, was an effective cure for bronchial conditions, asthma, congestive heart failure, colds/flu, chest congestion, and diarrhea.

In the seventh century the Prophet Muhammad proclaimed oregano as an effective cure for colds and flu, a fact which is proven today. He also said that it, along with other spices, such as frankincense, should be used in the home for fumigation. In addition, it was this man who was the inventor of natural perfumes for the body. What's more, Jesus was fond of aromatic oils and often perfumed his body, as did, apparently, Moses. It was Jesus who said that there could be nothing better than an aromatic, heat-producing ointment applied to the body. Too, the modern industry of perfumery, where the body is made fragrant with natural extracts from animals and plants, is attributed to him, since, clearly, it was through him that this was brought to the West. What's more, according to Wooten the entire field of essential oil medicine was brought to Europe through the efforts of the Islaamic peoples, who followed the Prophet's lead on popularizing distilled plant oils.

Regarding oregano-like plants Grieve has much to say. She quotes a number of Medieval herbalists, who greatly touted its powers. These herbalists proclaimed that the plants of this family, the wild types, which grow in the mountains, are entirely safe. She quotes Culpepper, who said that people should never worry about this hot oil, because it is entirely safe. The oil is, notes Grieve, a powerful antiseptic, yet, again, it is safe. It can even be taken daily, all these herbalists agree, with significant benefit.

Yet, what is the conclusion of modern science? Is there definite proof of its powers? What about safety? In fact, the safety is assured, and it can be taken with impunity. There is, perhaps, one exception. This is pregnant mothers, who should take it reasonably, like a few drops daily. When derived from the true wild oregano spice, it is merely oregano oil. Thus, it is a food extract and is harmless. Moreover, it is infinitely safer than many substances which pregnant women unthinkingly take such as aspartame, food dyes, sulfites, MSG, caffeine, and cola bean, all of which are, to a degree, poisonous.

Yet, in pregnancy there is usually no need to take large amounts. Instead, the whole crude herb can be taken on a daily basis and, if necessary, in significant amounts. A reasonable dosage for pregnant women of this supplement is four to six capsules daily. However, there is no harm in taking twice this amount, and this would be an appropriate dose for anyone suffering from poor nutrition or trace mineral deficiency. This form of wild oregano is exceedingly nourishing for pregnant women, since the whole crude herb is a top source of highly absorbable trace minerals such as chelated magnesium, calcium, phosphorus, zinc, and copper. As well, the oil—the true wild type derived from the edible whole spice (blue label brand)—can be rubbed topically on the body, on the soles of the feet and chest, as often as necessary to fight infection.

Animal studies

There have been a number of animal studies done on wild oregano. Premier of these was a study done by Manohar and Ingram published in *Molecular and Cellular Biochemistry* regarding the antifungal power of wild oregano oil. Here, mice were infected with a common human pathogen, *Candida albicans*. In the control group, given only olive oil, all the mice died. In the groups given either potent antifungal drugs or the oregano oil, virtually all the mice survived.

In this study in addition to natural wild oregano oil a synthetic type of oregano was given. Yet, while the synthetic oregano did kill the candida and saved the mice, even so, the mice after the treatment were sickly. In contrast, the mice treated with the true wild oregano oil were healthy and vigorous. The drug treated mice were also sickly appearing, because of the toxicity of synthetic chemicals. This was manifested by matting of the fur and sluggish behavior. The researchers concluded that the wild oregano oil is a potentially effective treatment for human candida infection and that it may well be effective, even for severe fungal/yeast infections.

Chaml and his group publishing in the *Brazilian Journal of Infectious Diseases* also studied the active ingredients of oil of wild oregano in rats. Here, too, the rats were infected with yeasts, that is candida. These rats had severely suppressed immune systems and were inoculated with the yeasts. Then, the rats were given the oregano's active ingredients. It was determined that the oregano treatment destroyed the fungi and prevented further invasion and that this treatment was more effective than antifungal drugs. While in the control group the yeast fully invaded the oral tissues, that is the tongue, and could not be destroyed. In contrast, in the oregano, that is carvacrol, treated group the fungus was completely obliterated. The conclusion was that the active ingredients of oil of wild oregano are potent antifungal agents against the candida yeasts that cause human infections.

These are significant results. In test tubes and petri dishes it is well known that oregano oil kills molds and fungi. Yet, here, it is proven that it does so in living beings. Furthermore, these studies demonstrate that the natural wild oil is superior to drugs in the treatment of experimental candidiasis. This is no minor issue. Rather, it is a landmark finding worthy of great press. Even so, relatively few people realize that this truly natural substance is more potent in the destruction of yeasts and fungi than any known drug. Nor are they aware that it is, unlike drugs, capable of destroying a wide range of such fungi.

It is not just yeasts and fungi that this natural substance destroys. This is because it is also a potent antibacterial agent. This, again, is proven primarily through animal studies. It was Preuss and Ingram who demonstrated that the wild oregano oil kills a wide range of noxious bacteria, including drug resistant forms. Here, mice were infected with penicillin-resistant staph and then either treated with a control substance, an antibiotic, that is Vancomycin, and wild oregano oil. The control mice all died, while half the Vancomycin and oregano oil treated mice survived. However, the researchers concluded that the oregano treated mice were healthier in appearance than the drug treated mice.

Some people say that this is of no consequence, this is just an animal study. Yet, what difference does it make? The point is that this natural cure, this wild oil of oregano, is superior to all drugs. Plus, such results are even confirmed by the U.S. government, which to a degree has resisted the truth about the powers of this substance. Thus, the confirmation by this entity is particularly impressive, seeing that wild oregano is regarded as a conflict of interest, that is regarding the pharmaceutical cartel. This is the issue upon which to concentrate. In fact, it is a spectacular result. Moreover, this is a highly relevant finding, because the same result occurred in humans, in this case a viral disease known as hepatitis C. Before describing the hepatitis C study consider the results of an in vitro (test tube) study of oil of wild oregano against the cold and flu viruses. In the study the virus was caused to infect chicken embryo cells to the degree of some 5,000,000 viruses per milliliter of fluid. Thus, there were hundreds of millions of viruses in the solution. The oregano oil was then added to the solution. Incredibly, in a mere 20 minutes over 99% of the viruses were destroyed and in one instance, in this case the cold virus versus a multiple spice extract, 100% of all viruses were killed.

A 100% kill in 20 minutes is a major feat. There is no drug available which can do so. With the flu virus it took a higher concentration to achieve a near 100% kill, some 10-times greater than that used against the cold virus. Yet, regardless, this is a stupendous result. It essentially defines a true cure for the common cold and flu.

The mechanism of action for this power has been proven. Apparently, the oil of wild oregano and similar heat-producing spice oils, such as oil of wild sage, cumin oil, clove oil, and cinnamon oil, shatter the viruses. It was Siddiqui publishing in *Medical Science Research* who demonstrated this on numerous cold-like viruses. He placed the viruses in petri dishes and added various spice oils, including oil of oregano and cinnamon, and then viewed this under the electron microscope. What he discovered was that the viruses were "disintegrated" a result he deemed "remarkable." Even so, there is no drug which can achieve this.

So, since wild oregano can destroy seasonal viruses, which are, generally, not regarded as major killers, what can it do against the real killer viruses such as the hepatitis viruses, particularly the deadly hepatitis C? A human trial conducted by Dr. Abdul Ghany proves that here, too, the spice oils are unmatched. In this trial some 14 people with hepatitis C, as manifested by high blood levels of the hepatitis C virus as well as liver enzymes, the latter being evidence of liver damage, were treated with high doses of oil of wild oregano. Some of these patients were also treated with natural wild flushing agents such as the total body purging agent. The results were exceptional, with the majority, 80%, showing significant improvement, which is evidence of the destruction of the virus.

Several cases showed a dramatic results, with complete clearance of the hepatitis C virus from the blood in two months, along with normalization of the liver enzymes. In one of these cases after two years treatment there was complete clearance, with viral titers being reduced from 5.5 million per centimeter of blood to virtually zero. This was despite the fact that the individual under treatment continued to drink wine. In her case as well as a result of the combined therapy of oil of wild oregano, high or super-strength variety plus the wild triple greens flushing agent, there was a dramatic normalization of liver enzyme levels. This means that the oregano/wild greens therapy normalized liver function. Again, there is no drug or even group of drugs which can achieve this. All these individuals were hopeless cases, where the standard medical treatment had failed.

This is no surprise. In 20 minutes in a study done by Microbiotest, reported in *Antiviral Research*, it was found that high dose oil of wild oregano obliterated virtually all traces of a tough strain of flu virus, killing hundreds of millions of viruses. In the same study a multiple spice complex, as well as the oil of wild oregano, decimated a variant of the bird flu, although a much higher dose, 25 times as high, was required. Thus, for any life-threatening viral infections, including infections by animal pathogens and hepatitis viruses, the regular normal dosage is insufficient. Incredibly, up to 25 or 30 times the normal dosages are necessary such as, for instance, 20 or 40 drops of the super strength form of wild oregano dozens of times daily and several multiple spice capsules five or ten times daily or even every hour. It is not a matter of whether or not it will work but is, rather, a matter of whether or not the person takes enough of these potent antiviral agents to make it work.

Antibacterial studies and more

People regard bacteria as particularly tough, since they are able to resist the most powerful drugs known. Yet, they are no match for oil of wild oregano. There are a number of studies which prove that the oil destroys bacteria. At Georgetown University it was found that it does so, even in bacterially infected mice, even if the mice are infected with drug resistant varieties. Here, as mentioned previously the wild oregano oil saved the animals' lives. Again, at Georgetown it was discovered that in the petri dish wild oregano oil, using the well known national brand, obliterates five disease-causing bacteria, which are staph, klebsiella, E. coli, a variant of the TB bacillus known as *Mycobacterium terrae*, and the anthrax bacillus. In contrast, no antibiotic is capable of killing such a wide range of bacteria. With the various work done by this university on bacteria it was concluded that the wild oregano oil is likely a "useful antimicrobial agent" for the "prevention and therapy" of bacterial infections. This is a major statement by an orthodox university in an arena which clamors for so-called definitive scientific proof.

In 2004 in *Applied and Environmental Microbiology* Lin and his group showed that the growth of a very powerful bacteria, *Listeria monocytes*, was blocked by a combination of oregano and cranberry extracts. Listeria is a major cause of food poisoning from, for instance, contaminated luncheon meats and cheese. This combination is available as a wild cranberry/oregano flushing agent taken as drops under the tongue. The typical dose for bladder, urinary, and intestinal disorders, including diarrhea, is 20 drops three times daily.

Italian investigators publishing in the *Italian Journal of Food Science* found that oregano oil is active against another food poisoning bacteria: E. coli. The type of E. coli they tested against was no minor bacteria but rather was the most dangerous, mutated type, which is E. coli O157:H7. This is a cause of potentially terminal bloody diarrhea plus kidney failure. Globally, yearly, this bacteria kills thousands of people. The Italian study proved that the oregano oil destroyed this form of E. coli. A mere half percent of the oil added to the bacterial solution was sufficient to kill virtually all bacteria.

Investigators in Poland publishing in *Current Medicinal Chemistry* investigated the antibacterial powers of a variety of spice oils. While they determined that oils of oregano and thyme were most powerful some 30 different bacteria, along with 9 different fungi, were found to be killed or inhibited by essential oil therapy.

Greek investigators confirmed in particular the antibacterial and antifungal powers of the wild oil. These researchers publishing in *Acta Horticulturae* found that compared to other plant oils the essential oil of oregano was most potent as a germicide against both noxious bacteria and molds. Incredibly, the oil obliterated cultures of E. coli, pseudomonas, bacillus, and *Aspergillus niger*. Pseudomonas is a cause of drug-resistant infections and a highly fatal type of pneumonia. E. coli readily causes diarrhea as well as a type of kidney failure. Aspergillus causes severe lung infections as well as asthma. Thus, any such disease caused by these germs is readily cured by the Mediterranean-source wild oregano. Interestingly, these investigators studied two types of wild oil of oregano. This was both the steam distilled extract and the carbon dioxide (super-critical) extract. In all investigations they found the steam distilled extract, the type primarily recommended in this book, to be the most potent as a germ killer.

In another study done in London and published in the *World Journal of Gastroenterology* the growth of the notorious human pathogen, H. pylori, was blocked or destroyed by spices. Using a boiled extract of turmeric, oregano, cumin, and ginger, among other 'foods', were found to be active against this organism. This correlates with the findings of a major maker of spice oil extracts, where four humans suffering with H. pylori infection were tested. These individuals were given capsules of multiple spice extract, containing dessicated oils of oregano, cumin, sage, and cinnamon. The results were promising. Using a test known as the breath urea test, which is a marker for H. pylori activity—the organism produces urea, which can be measured in the breath—it was found that the daily intake of six capsules of multiple spice complex, two with each meal, resulted in an 80% reduction in breath urea levels. This occurred in only two weeks. This means that the multiple spice complex destroyed the H. pylori in humans. This explains why in countless cases in humans there is a great improvement in symptoms through the wild spice therapy.

It is no surprise that the spice oils can achieve this. These are highly potent germicides. In a study done in Greece it was found that in particular oil of wild oregano is an exceptional antibacterial agent, even in tiny quantities. The study published in the *Journal of Agricultural Research* determined that a mere one in 50,000 dilution was sufficient to inhibit the growth of bacteria, while a one in 4,000 dilution caused virtual complete destruction of the germs. The bacteria against which this tiny amount of wild oil of oregano proved effective included staph, salmonella, E. coli, and pseudomonas, the latter being notoriously difficult to kill. Regarding the latter any substance which can kill pseudomonas is an exceptional one. The degree of power was dependent upon the type of oregano used, with the wild high mountain varieties being most powerful. The investigators also determined, incredibly, that the wild oregano oil was also highly active against human cancer cells, which were destroyed by the oregano in culture.

It is well known that E. coli kills. It also causes vast human disability. It is a major cause of dire infections in hospitalized patients and readily infects the blood, intestines, and kidneys. Yet, in nature there is an obvious cure for this, which is the wild oil of oregano. In the Netherlands a study was done demonstrating the vast powers of oil of oregano against this germ. Published in *Letters in Applied Microbiology*, 2002, this destructive power was clearly shown, when researchers found that oil of oregano completely destroys this pathogen, a fact also confirmed at Georgetown University. The Dutch study demonstrated that the oregano was "successful in killing" massive numbers of E. coli, with "no viable cells recovered." Yet, this all occurred in less than a minute.

Can anyone fathom it? The wild oregano oil, a natural product, obliterates this pathogen. What's more, it does so in the human body, plus it achieves this without any harm. This is a monumental discovery, fully equivalent to the discovery of penicillin, rather, far more so. Actually, there is no comparison for the two. Penicillin only kills bacteria and then only a few types. In contrast, oregano oil destroys virtually every bacteria known and also kills viruses, molds, fungi, and parasites. There is no drug nor any group of drugs, which are comparable. This is why this discovery is so revolutionary.

Again, consider it. The wild oil of oregano destroys bacteria, fungi, molds, viruses, mites, and parasites. In contrast, a single antibiotic may only be able to kill, for instance, a few species of bacteria or fungi. An antibiotic is never effective against all bacteria or fungi. Yet, the high mountain oil of wild Mediterranean source—this destroys virtually all species of bacteria and fungi plus essentially all viruses, and thousands of such species.

The discovery of the vast powers of this oil is an exceptional breakthrough. It is a major breakthrough because, through this great knowledge, a great number of lives will be saved. In fact, even a modest awareness regarding the wild oregano oil, with, now, minor millions currently using it, has saved countless lives, while preventing much misery. With drugs, those who make even a miniscule discovery of such a degree are given great accolades. Where is the great praise for the discovery of the oil of wild oregano? The major press is virtually silent regarding this. There are no documentaries revealing this discovery, informing the people of its diverse benefits. This is a true medical breakthrough, yet, unlike the discovery of penicillin the world at-large doesn't know about it. This is the most ludicrous circumstance that can be conceived.

Even so, what does this reveal? It demonstrates the great power of the master of this universe, that this grand Being could produce a single plant, which has the power to obliterate dangerous germs. Moreover, regarding this antiseptic power this is not merely against one species of such germs but rather against virtually all species. Furthermore, it does so without the least side effects.

Parasites, too, succumb to spice oils. The various spice oils and their extracts are the primary antiseptic agents known. For instance, thymol has long been used as a purging agent for parasites. It was once the major medicine listed in the original medical books, from the early 1800s until about 1950, for killing parasites. The active ingredient of oregano is carvacrol, which is similar to thymol. A human study published in *Phytotherapy Research* was performed on oregano oil versus parasites, in this instance the intestinal amebas *Entamoeba hartmanni* and *Endolimax nana* as well as the protozoan *Blastocystis hominis*. In this study 14 patients with proven intestinal infection by these parasites were given capsules of oregano oil in an emulsion. The results were highly positive, with complete destruction of the parasites achieved in eight of the patients. Moreover, regarding those who tested positive for *Blastocystis hominis* through the oral oregano therapy gastrointestinal symptoms improved in seven of the 11 cases.

Other spice oils which exhibit potent antiparasitic powers include oil of clove bud, oil of cumin, oil of sage, and oil of juniper. Thus, in addition to the oil of oregano a multiple spice extract is indicated for the destruction of deep seated parasitic infections. For such significant parasitic infestations, again, the oregano oil alone may not be sufficient. From the same high grade maker the individual may also find single oils which have additional anti-parasitic power, such as oils of cumin, fennel, and clove, or, perhaps, a combination of these. Also, consider the intake of raw pumpkin seeds, which may be taken simultaneously with the various spice oils.

The mold crisis: scientific proof

Molds are a vast cause of human disease. In this regard the diseases they cause are far more extensive than previously realized. It is now being demonstrated that common molds found in damp places or even dry environments actually cause disease. In some instances the diseases/syndromes may be dangerous, even potentially fatal. These diseases and syndromes, now proven to be caused in part by molds, include the following:

- acute sinusitis
- chronic sinusitis
- rhinitis, including allergic rhinitis
- bronchitis
- repeated bouts of pneumonia
- pulmonary fibrosis
- asthma
- pleurisy
- mis-diagnosed lung cancer
- chronic fatigue syndrome
- fibromyalgia
- intestinal inflammation
- persistent nose bleeds
- chronic earaches

This is an extensive list. Now, the mystery behind these diseases and conditions is largely revealed. In order for there to be relief from these conditions the molds must be destroyed. This is through the intake of the wild oregano whole herb, along with *Rhus coriaria,* as well as the oil of wild oregano. In addition, regarding sinus infestation a wild-oregano-based nasal mist with oil of wild bay leaf, oil of wild sage, and natural sea salt is potent. The molds in the sinuses are deep-seated, and, thus, such a spray is an essential component of the therapy.

Regarding the fungal/mold connection to sinus and other respiratory disorders there is extensive evidence. In 1999 Mayo as published in *Mayo Clinic Proceedings* investigated the causes behind sinusitis in 100 cases. All these patients were resistant to standard therapies, including antibiotics and surgery. The nasal and sinus membranes were washed by gavage, and the resultant secretions were cultured. In all cases the molds and fungi were found to be the causative factors. No invasive bacteria were found. This is stark proof that for disorders of the respiratory tract invasion by fungi and molds are the first consideration. It also demonstrates that common molds are highly invasive and that they readily cause human disease.

Both black and green molds readily infect the sinus cavities. This infection may create a great degree of disability. It may act as a kind of focus of infection, resulting in chronic disease. Diseases which may be caused in part by fungal sinusitis include bronchitis, pneumonia, migraines, asthma, chronic fatigue syndrome, gastritis, esophagitis, and fibromyalgia.

Wild oregano: a cancer fighter?

There is also significant antitumor properties of oil of wild oregano. This was proven by Greek investigators, who showed that oil of wild oregano destroys cancer cells in solution. In this study, published in the *Journal of Agricultural Food Chemistry,* investigators merely put the oregano oil in a solution with four different human cancer cell lines. In all four in a mere dilution of 1 to 4000 the oregano killed all cancerous cells.

Turkish investigators have investigated the anticancer properties further. Here, it was discovered that in children with leukemia oregano, as both the watery steam-extracted essence, that is the juice, and the steam-extracted oil, were effective in inducing remission. The children with this disease treated with oregano improved significantly compared to those not treated with the spice extracts. Yet, many might ask, how does oregano, a mere spice, help reverse this dreaded disease?

A study performed in India by Srihari and colleagues may explain the mechanism. In this study rats were exposed to a coal tar-derived cancer-causing chemical. The chemical induces colon cancer in the rats. Also, the chemical causes chemical changes, leading to the cancers. These chemical changes are known as free radical generation. These free radicals readily cause genetic cancer, which can then lead to cancer. The free radicals can be measured in the tissues of the rats after they are sacrificed. High levels are a signal of the potential for the development of tumors. In the control rats given the coal tar derivative the levels of free radicals were high. However, in the rats given this carcinogen, who were also given daily doses of oregano, there was a reversal of this toxicity; the levels of free radicals were low. Furthermore, while in the control rats the levels of protective or anticancer enzymes, such as glutathione reductase, catalase, and superoxide dismutase, were low in the oregano treated rats the levels were virtually normal. This, the investigators concluded, "suggested (an) anti-cancer property of oregano."

An even more compelling study was published by researchers in Florida. Cancer, the researchers knew, is associated with disorders in blood clotting. The cancer causes the blood to thicken, which impedes both the blood flow and the immune system. Also, this thickening makes it easier for the cancer to grow and, particularly, to metastasize. This is because with thick blood the cancer cells can easily be transported from one region to another, whereas thin blood favors the inhibition of cancer growth. The agent involved in the thickening of the blood is thrombin, which is found in higher than normal levels in cancer victims. The researchers, publishing in the journal *Fitoterapia,* found that substances in the oregano plant actually block thrombin. This means that the oregano is a natural blood regulator, perhaps a mild thinning agent. Yet, this thinning or, rather, normalization property is never dangerous. No one bleeds abnormally from wild oregano. What's more, topically, the oil has the opposite effect, because on wounds it helps speed clotting. Thus, again the action of this invaluable substance is to bring normality to the tissues.

The researchers isolated the blood clotting-regulating substances from the oregano, which are aristolochic acid and D-raffinose. In addition, the power of these substances was tested against leukemia cells, which also thrive among high thrombin levels. Again, thick blood favors the development of leukemia. The conclusion of the researchers was compelling, which is that these components of wild oregano, particularly aristolochic acid, are *'confirmed* to possess activity against cancer.' Aristocholic acid is found in the whole ground herb, which may be purchased as capsules, along with its companion herb *Rhus coriaria*, or bulk powder.

Too, for defeating cancer the power of the immune system is crucial. The white blood cells must be in a high state of activity in order to cleanse the body of this disease. The immune-boosting power of wild oregano is massive. Both the oil and the crude wild herb greatly enhance the immune system. Moreover, they do so to a degree far greater than any other natural substance. This has been confirmed in a number of studies.

Perhaps the most compelling is a study done by Polish investigators. Here, publishing in *Herba Polonica*, the investigators studied some 33 herbs for their capacity to increase the levels of interferon, a key marker for immune activity. Interferon is a protein produced by white blood cells in the fight against infection. Low levels of this substance mean that the immune system is failing to adequately combat the infection/disease. Of all herbs tested only the wild oregano significantly increased interferon levels. In Germany in an animal study oregano was proven to directly increase white blood cell function. Investigators concluded that this herb/spice had a general immune boosting effect as manifested by an increase in germ killing lymphocytes in both the bloodstream and within the lymph glands.

What does this reveal? It reveals that the wild oregano fits the body system perfectly and that it enhances the body's protective mechanisms. In contrast, drugs function to poison the body's mechanisms in order to control or alter symptoms. The mechanisms and results of these two therapies are entirely different. With the wild oregano the healing powers of the body are enhanced. With drugs, these powers are corrupted.

More proof: antioxidant and anticancer powers

As mentioned previously extracts of wild oregano kill tumor cells. Thus, these extracts act as a kind of natural chemotherapy against cancerous growths. This killing effect is because of the antiseptic powers of these extracts but may also be related to their profound antioxidant powers.

Regarding the direct killing power this, again, may be related to the killing of germs. German investigators have determined that a majority of cancers are infested with yeasts and molds, which may act to a degree to cause the tumors. By killing these yeasts and molds the cancers involute. Also, a number of investigators have demonstrated that tumors are largely caused by viruses. This is true of brain tumors, bone cancer, breast cancer, and sarcomas. Viruses are also implicated in leukemia and lymphoma. Thus, obviously, the destruction of such viruses will lead to the destruction of the tumor.

There have been a number of human cases, where large doses of the oil of wild oregano, Mediterranean-source, along with the essence/juice of wild oregano, have obliterated tumors. In humans elimination of cancerous growths have been seen in cases of prostate, bladder, pancreatic, and tongue cancer. There has also been reversal of cancerous growths/tissue in cases of lymphoma and leukemia. This has been confirmed by careful physical and biochemical examination.

As proven by CT scan and MRI the tumors, which were previously diagnosed, have simply disappeared. This is because of the destructive powers of the wild oregano extracts against both the tumor cells and the various germs which inhabit them. The germs develop a symbiotic relationship with the cancer cells. When the germs are killed, the cancer cells are defenseless. So, they, too, die. This destruction process is enhanced through the use of wild raw berry extracts (for more information see the *Wild Berry Cure*, same author, Knowledge House Publishers).

It is no surprise that such natural extracts are antitumor. This would be expected based on the plethora of research regarding such natural extracts. For instance, mere berries, if unaltered or freeze-dried, have significant antitumor properties. Even so, medical authorities resist such a statement and even would fight it. This is despite the fact that the science which demonstrates this effect is medical. For instance, in humans as demonstrated by Ohio State's Gary Stoner black raspberry is effective in destroying tumor cells.

Other investigators have demonstrated that extracts of cranberry exhibit significant antitumor properties. In addition, cranberry extract greatly improved the efficacy of orthodox treatments such as chemotherapy.

As well, people who promote or recommend such substances are often attacked or condemned. Even so, while this is not an attempt to promote a cure for cancer there is a simple fact which cannot be denied. This is the fact that natural substances, including high potency extracts of wild oregano and wild raw berry extracts, efficiently kill tumor cells and do so as effectively as standard drugs.

Regarding cancer and other degenerative diseases there are a number of other bases for wild oregano's impressive powers. This relates to the antioxidant powers of this potent spice. Compared to other plants wild oregano scores exceedingly high in antioxidative powers, far higher than most fruit and vegetables and also higher than virtually all other spices. Only two common substances scored higher than the oregano, which are propolis and clove.

A test was performed to evaluate how this antioxidant power impacts cancer. This was done on fruit flies, which were subjected to toxic stress. The stress causes mutations. The flies which were given the oregano oil had no increase in mutations, so this demonstrated that oregano had no carcinogenic effects. However, the real test was to see if the oregano oil had positive effects, which it did. This was because the oil "strongly inhibited" the ability of the toxin, in this case urethane, to cause mutations in the genes.

The researchers sought to determine the mechanism of just how the oregano oil could protect the genes. They determined that the oil, notably its active ingredient carvacrol, directly protected the genes from urethane-induced free radical damage.

This is confirmed by the work of Srihari and his group, who tested oregano as an antioxidant in the fight against colon cancer. Here, researchers used an oregano extract to combat the cancer-causing effects of a petrochemical derivative known as DMH (dimethylhydrazine). The DMH was fed to rats, and the expected result is massive free radical formation in the rat colon, a precursor to cancer. As mentioned previously in the control rats the level of free radicals, measured as peroxides, rose massively. In contrast, in the oregano-treated rats there was no such rise. What's more, the oregano treatment caused an increase in the production of highly protective antioxidant enzymes. In other words, the oregano caused the rats' bodies to produce protective compounds. This proves that rather than any possible harm from this spice there is only benefit. Furthermore, the protection is exceedingly potent to such a degree that the noxious effects of cancer-causing chemicals is neutralized.

This indicates a significant fact. It is that not taking the oregano therapy is dangerous, because, without exception, this is a highly protective spice. This is true, even in exceedingly fatal diseases.

There is yet another proof that is exceedingly impressive. Anyone who would ignore this surely is troubled. This is the fact that wild oregano is a regenerative substance. This regenerative power is real proof of the blessed nature of this spice rather its divine nature.

Again, this is a mere natural wild spice, which has all such properties. In contrast, there is no modern medical treatment which is even remotely similar to its powers and diversity. Yet, how could it be? Such a potent substance not only reverses disease, not only prevents it, but also revives all cells. This proves that the divinely made medicines, as whole foods, are infinitely more powerful than drugs. It could be no accident. It is incredible but true: while man-made chemicals, including drugs, destroy tissue, even critical internal organs, wild oregano regenerates them. In the study the intent was to evaluate oregano oil, more specifically its main active ingredient carvacrol, upon the regenerative capacity of the liver. This was after the liver in test animals was partially removed (70%), a procedure known as hepatectomy. Normally, this would lead to disruption of all functions, and regeneration is slow.

The effect of the oregano was easy to measure. The livers were simply weighed before and after treatment. Only one dose of the oregano extract was given. Incredibly, this single dose alone caused a significant increase in rate of liver cell regeneration compared to controls. This is final proof that the oregano is not only entirely safe and that it is also required for those who seek optimal health. It is also clearly a most potent substance for preventing disease and, as well, for, perhaps, exceeding lifespan.

The power for increasing lifespan is obvious. Mediterranean-source high-mountain oregano extracts achieve this through a variety of capacities, as follows:

- the quenching of noxious free radicals, which accelerate the aging process
- the neutralization of cancer-causing toxic chemicals, including coal tar and petrochemical derivatives
- the stimulation in the production of various enzymes, which help halt or reverse the aging process, including glutathione peroxidase, glutathione reductase, superoxide dismutase, and peroxidase

- the destruction of deep-seated germs, which cause chronic degenerative diseases
- the prevention of serious or life-threatening infection through the daily intake (of both the wild oregano oil and the crude herb combined with *Rhus coriaria,* garlic, and onion)
- the neutralization of potentially life-threatening allergic reactions, including reactions to peanuts, drugs, and shrimp and also the neutralization of venom from bees, snakes, scorpions, spiders, and similar creatures
- the direct antioxidant function, which helps preserve all cells against the aging process

Biting bugs: spice oils to the rescue

Spice oils are natural bug repellents. Testing proves their power. The spice oils in specific combinations have been demonstrated to be virtually equal in effectiveness to common chemical repellents and in some cases superior to such repellents.

In Canada at the University of Guelph testing was done on one such repellent, which is a combination of several spice oils. These spice oils included wild oils of oregano, bay leaf, and lavender oil plus nutmeg oil (and possibly basil oil). In this test a box was filled with mosquitoes and the volunteers' arms were put in the box. The arms of volunteers were sprayed with the herbal bug repellent, known as Herbal Bug-X. For an hour there was full repellent effects. Moreover, when this herbal formula was taken internally, since it is entirely edible, even here there was modest repellent effects. This is significant. It means that even if the spice extracts are taken internally, still, they exert a significant degree of repellent effects.

This repellent has been tested in the deep bush. This is in northern Canada, where the biting insects are fierce. Here, test subjects have achieved at least two hours of repellent effects with the spice oil spray. In order to increase this repellent effect merely repeat the application. Yet, this is aromatic spice oils, which may be sprayed on the body as frequently as desired. Thus, this is a safe way to gain the same results as DEET and other carcinogenic repellents. The herbal spray is safe for infants and children as well as pets.

How to take wild oregano

The most important issue for taking wild oregano is to be sure to procure the truly wild type, which is hand-picked in the high mountains of the Mediterranean. The oregano can be taken in a number of ways. The ideal way is as drops under the tongue. Of course, this is hot. Some people are unable to tolerate this. In these cases it may be taken by mouth. Here, it can be merely swallowed and then followed with water or juice. Or it can be directly added to the water or juice and then swallowed.

It can also be put in food. For instance, it can be added to yogurt or drizzled on cheese. The oregano oil can also be added to cooking; in fact, cooking does not significantly weaken its powers. It should simply be added toward the end of any cooking, that is in stir fry, tomato sauces, and soup.

The oregano oil can be used as a meat rub. This is particularly valuable when cooking poultry, as it not only tenderizes the meat but it also kills noxious germs, which typically contaminate this food. Also, it may be added in small amounts to marinades and salad dressings.

The key is to consume it in any way possible. The person needs to, somehow, get it into the system on a regular basis. This is highly protective against all sudden infections as well as a variety of chronic diseases. There are also gelatin capsules. These are highly convenient and may be taken in large doses. For those who seek vegetable gelatin there are multiple spice complex capsules in pine tree-based gelatin.

There is also the watery essence or juice. This is a highly easy type of oregano to consume. It is merely a matter of drinking it. For those who do not like the taste it can be added to tomato, carrot, or V-8 juice. Or, it may be taken straight. It may also be added to grapefruit juice. Orange juice tends to be too sweet for the oregano essence and tends to neutralize some of its powers.

The crude whole herb, combined with *Rhus coriaria,* is another convenient form. Surely, the capsules can be swallowed, but they can also be opened and the contents sprinkled over food. This wild oregano complex makes an ideal additive for eggs, quiche, and yogurt. It may also be sprinkled over cheese. As well, it is excellent in marinades and stir fry. This crude herbal formula is also available as a bulk supplement. This is the ideal form for using in food. The bulk formula contains a spoon. A scoop or two per day added to food or juice is an ideal daily dose. Note: this makes a luscious additive to pizza, marinara sauce, and spaghetti.

Another issue is the occasional complaint of the spicy nature of wild oregano oil. The crushed herbal capsules may also be too spicy for some people. Thus, certain people complain that these natural medicines "repeat" on them. This is easily remedied, since this usually results from taking the wild oregano on an empty stomach, which can result in belching. All that is necessary to eliminate this is to take it with a full meal. Ideally, this should be a meal rich in natural fat such as the fats of meat, poultry, whole milk products, and fatty vegetables, like olives and avocados. Even so, if a person would just persist in taking it on an empty stomach, eventually, this repeating stops, and it is well tolerated.

Again, wild oregano is spicy. This may be an issue for people with weak hearts and high blood pressure. Even so, oregano is good for the heart and arteries. Yet, to prevent any supposed reaction for people with these conditions the oregano should be taken with full meals, and the meal should contain fat.

Occasionally, the aggressive use of oil of wild oregano may raise blood pressure. While this is a temporary reaction this is due to the capacity of the oregano to increase the pumping power of the heart. The way to avoid this is to take the oregano with a full meal that is rich in fat. Or, a drop or two can be mixed in a tablespoon or two of extra virgin olive oil and taken directly in grapefruit juice or lemon juice.

For some people a thick juice is the only way that the oregano oil is tolerated, that is for daily consumption. Such thick juices include tomato, V-8, pear, peach, apricot, and carrot juice. Or, another option for the person who can't handle the taste is to take the gelatin capsules. A reasonable daily dose is one or two capsules twice daily. Whenever taking daily doses of oregano (more than five or ten drops daily) it is a good idea to also take a probiotic or, perhaps, eat natural full fat yogurt regularly.

Again, regarding side effects there is a reaction, which is possible. This is the reaction of cleansing. Here, the oregano is actually killing noxious germs, but the body is revealing this. Thus, symptoms may rarely develop, especially in people who are highly toxic or who have intestinal overgrowth of noxious germs. The oregano may cause diarrhea—because the person's gut is too overloaded with parasites and other pathogens, and these pathogens begin to fight back, thus, the diarrhea. There is rarely some bloating. All this is good. The secret is to continue the oregano therapy or, actually, increase the dosage, not to pull back. Even so, with the crude herbal capsules plus *Rhus coriaria* symptoms such as these are rare, as this is the most mild form of oregano to consume.

As mentioned previously there may also be flu-like symptoms. This, too, is a good sign. It means that the immune system is fighting and, in fact, destroying the organism and that perhaps the germ, too, is fighting. Yet, the germs are losing this fight, and the key is to continue the battle, never withdrawing the dose until the cure is achieved.

The topical power of wild oregano

Oil of wild oregano is a potent natural medicine with a wide range of powers. One of its greatest curative effects relates to its topical use. The highly aromatic oil can be vigorously rubbed on the body. It can even be scrubbed into the tissues. Here, it is a massive activator of the lymphatic system. It also activates the local or surface circulation, in other words, it boosts blood flow to the skin. This is critical, since the skin is the largest organ in the body.

Because the skin is large it is also vulnerable. In other words it may be readily attacked. A number of creatures can attack and infect it. Yet other creatures inject the skin with venom, some of which can prove fatal. Wild oregano oil is a lifesaver in all such circumstances. This is because it is a potent antivenom as well as antiseptic. It is also highly destructive against mites, fleas, lice, and various other parasites, which may attack the skin, hair, and scalp. Whenever there is any insult against the skin the oil of oregano is the treatment of choice. It is a potent antiinflammatory agent but also a powerful antihistamine. It is a germicide and also a miticide. It is also a larvacide. Regarding any sudden parasite, which attacks the skin, the oregano oil will kill it. It is powerful, because it deeply penetrates the skin, where it creates heat and therefore eases inflammation. This oil is one of the most potent antivenoms known. It effectively neutralizes spider, snake, bee, and scorpion venom as well as the venom from various sea creatures. Thus, it is the number one natural medicine to have available in all peoples' medicine chests. It should be applied vigorously to any venomous bite. As a result, all danger from such bite will be eliminated.

Despite its high heat production for open wounds the oil is also ideal. In particular, it is invaluable for contaminated wounds, particularly bites. This includes dog, cat, and human bites. All such bites may cause deep-seated infections, which may then result in chronic disease. These risks can be eliminated through the use of the wild oregano oil, which should be repeatedly applied to the wound/bite site and should also be taken orally or sublingually.

Oregano oil is an excellent medicine for burns. This is true of all types of burns. Rapidly, it reduces the swelling and inflammation in burns and should, ideally, be used both topically and internally.

A person may find it bizarre that such a hot, spicy oil is an ideal burn remedy. Yet, it is as if like treats like. The oregano oil is, for instance, far more powerful in reversing the pain and damage of burns than the more mild oil lavender.

Yet, lavender is touted for burns, while no one is aware of the greatness in this regard of oregano oil. For sunburns there is no better remedy than this oil. Lavender oil is also effective and, perhaps, the two can be used together. The oregano oil should be applied immediately to any sunburned region and then applied repeatedly, especially in severe cases. For a more mild treatment, which is also effective, use the wild oregano cream, which contains additional powerful anti-burn oils such as wild lavender oil, wild St. John's wort oil, and Canadian balsam plus raw honey and propolis. This raw and completely natural cream is a highly effective burn treatment and has been used successfully on severe burns, including chemical burns.

This is demonstrated by a specific case, where a woman burned the palms of her hands with drain cleaner. Surely, without a miracle her hands would be hopelessly scarred. Realizing the powers of the wild oregano oil she had available the aforementioned oregano-based cream. Repeatedly, she applied this and essentially prevented permanent damage. In this regard it is well known that all the ingredients of this cream, that is wild oils of oregano, lavender, and St. John's wort, along with honey, propolis, and Canadian balsam, are all highly effective in healing burns.

Also, in the case of inflamed skin—the skin of psoriasis and eczema—an oregano-based essential oil cream is a boon. This is more soothing than the oil itself, and therefore it lends itself to healing damaged tissue. The cream readily penetrates into the skin with no residue. When applied to psoriatic and eczematous lesions, there is a temporary burning sensation then a sensation of cooling. There have been numerous cases of people with psoriasis and eczema who have seen their lesions improve and even disappear through the use of the cream. However, to achieve this it must be used regularly, and for difficult cases over a relatively prolonged period such as two or more months. The cream is also effective against bacteria and fungal infections of the skin such as acne, impetigo, ringworm, and athlete's foot. It may also be used for jock itch, that is if the person can withstand the temporary burning. Additionally, it is effective against rosacea, although for this condition in addition to this topical treatment the oregano oil, along with the whole crude herb, plus *Rhus coriaria*, should be taken internally. This is because rosacea is largely caused by infestation of the gut, particularly H. pylori infection of the stomach wall.

Even so, the most common use for oil of oregano topically is fungal infection. This includes toenail fungus, fingernail fungus, athlete's foot, jock itch, dandruff, and ringworm. For athlete's foot its effectiveness is unmatched. The same is true for ringworm. Diluted with extra virgin olive oil about one to 10, it also reverses jock itch. Regarding toenail fungus there have been a number of reports of benefit. This is usually through a combination of internal and external treatment. According to these reports the regular use leads to the destruction of the deep-seated fungal infestation, and within about three to six months the re-growth of a normal nail. These reports are unconfirmed. However, there is some basis for this. According to a preliminary report by Georgetown University, Washington, D. C., the wild oregano oil in a high strength form obliterated all traces of foot and toenail fungi. This was a test tube study, which will soon be followed with a human trial. The oil which was used is the original type supplied by a maker of the highest integrity. This is the spice oil of oregano, which is steam extracted from the hand-picked wild Mediterranean oregano leaves. It is the same oil of oregano used by the federal government in its research.

How to use wild oregano for pets

Wild oregano is a highly safe food/spice. It is easy to demonstrate its safety. Everyone knows that canaries are highly sensitive to toxins. These birds were formerly placed in mines as a means to act as a warning of toxic fumes. If the canary died, then, the miners were alerted to the potential for danger.

People who raise canaries are major users of oil of wild oregano. They use it to keep their birds healthy. In particular, they use it to prevent respiratory infections, which in such birds is usually fatal. In one instance the owner of a Florida song bird company was stricken with a dire circumstance: about one-third of her canaries were dying of respiratory ailments. Upon learning of the antifungal and antiviral powers of oil of wild oregano (hand-picked Mediterranean, original brand) the proprietor added this oil, a drop or two, into the canaries' water. This eliminated the crisis, and she no longer lost birds to sudden respiratory illness.

People often wonder how to use the oil for cats and dogs. This is relatively simple. The oil can merely be rubbed on their paws, then, of course, they will get it internally by licking it off. Also, the oregano may be sprayed on the underbelly, from which it will be absorbed systemically. As well, the crude herbal complex as a bulk powder can be added to all wet food.

The wild oregano-based spray may be used to deodorize the dog stench as well as cat litter boxes. Like pigs, dogs have no sweat glands and, thus, exude significant odor. While the owners may not realize it all others notice this canine smell in homes or vehicles inhabited by dogs. These regions can to a degree be deodorized largely by the regular use of spice oil sprays. Plus, the aroma of such sprays helps protect pets from pests such as fleas and ticks. As well, the dog's hide can be sprayed and therefore decontaminated.

The wild oregano spray contains oils of wild oregano, bay leaf, and lavender. These are emulsified into a creamy water. Sprayed on a dog or cat it acts as a flea repellent. It is also a minor tick repellent and is particularly effective as a mosquito repellent.

For killing ticks the oregano oil in a super- or high-strength form is most effective. Simply saturate a ball of cotton with the oregano oil, and hold over the tick. Do this until the tick dies, and then remove it. Then, after the tick is removed saturate another piece of cotton with the oregano oil, and tape it to the bite site. Leave this intact for 24 hours and remove. This should sterilize the site and prevent any spread of disease.

Birds benefit greatly from wild oregano. This is because these creatures are vulnerable to infections of the lungs, including various types of avian flu. The most vulnerable are caged birds, which can readily develop potentially fatal viral, bacterial, and/or fungal infections. For caged birds the oil of oregano, ideally the mycelized type, can be added to the water, about a drop per water tray. Also, the wild oregano-based spray may be used to decontaminate the cages or for purifying the air in aviaries.

Vaccines or oregano: which is superior?

There is no comparison between the oregano and vaccines. Oregano kills germs, while vaccines fail to do so. No one is killed by oregano, while vaccines cause countless fatalities. Vaccines cause brain damage; oregano boosts the function of the brain. Furthermore, while these injections actually cause in children immune depression, allergies, asthma, arthritis, and diabetes, all these diseases are completely prevented, as well as reversed, by the wild oregano. In addition, oregano oil, as well as the crude whole herb, eliminates childhood eczema, while in contrast vaccines cause this condition. So, how can they be compared? The fact is the wild oregano is incomparably more powerful—as well as infinitely more safe—than vaccines. In particular, the oil of oregano kills virtually all known viruses, while vaccines not only fail to kill viruses but also introduce dangerous viruses to the body. Thus, while the oregano obliterates illnesses vaccines actually cause them.

A parent will often says, "But if I don't vaccinate, aren't I putting my child's life at risk?" Yet, consider the actual facts. What is the number one cause for parents' reports to the government of sudden illness in children? It is exclusively vaccination. Also, vaccines are the number one cause of parents' reports of sudden death in a child. Compare this to the wild oregano oil, original type (blue label). There is not even a single case of a parent reporting the oregano as a cause of illness, even a minor illness, to the government, let alone fatality. The government even admits this, in other words, there are no complaints against the oregano. Yet, every year in the United States and Canada there are tens of thousands of such cases, children who were previously healthy and who were suddenly and direly sickened as a result of vaccination, reported by parents, including reports of hundreds of fatalities. Yes, vaccines kill, while wild oregano actually does the opposite, dramatically saving human lives.

So, people should investigate the dangers of vaccines. This is through doing research on the internet or in the library.

There are also books, which expound upon the great danger of these injections. One such book, the *Cause for Cancer Revealed* (Knowledge House Publishers, same author) exposes the cancer-causing role of vaccinations.

Common questions with wild oregano therapy

There are a number of questions which people frequently ask regarding the use of natural medicines. Often, people are concerned about how long a powerful-tasting substance, like the oil of oregano, can be used. Such people may be concerned about potential side effects, even though, for instance, oil of wild oregano is a food extract. There is also the concern regarding the great germicidal power of the wild oregano, that is in relation to the delicate natural bacteria in the intestines. Others are concerned that there may be poisonous effects of long-term intake or that there could be noxious results from killing pathogens, which is known as "die-off."

People may also be concerned about the potential for interactions with medications. Other people ask when should the oregano be taken, and can it be taken on an empty stomach, or is it preferable to take it with meals. All these are legitimate issues. Yet, perhaps the most compelling of these is simply how much should a person take and for how long should it be taken?

Regarding the regular use of the wild oregano, including the potent oil, this is a non-issue. It may be used on a daily basis in a reasonable amount, like three to five drops twice daily. This is for a relatively healthy person for maintenance. Regarding a person with an illness more can readily be taken, for instance, five to 20 drops or even greater amounts. Moreover, this can be taken daily until the condition is resolved. There are no toxic or side effects to such intake. The only side effect is the possibility of so-called die-off. Here, a person may experience temporary effects, such as tiredness and muscle aches, which is the result of killing large amounts of pathogens. These effects can be eliminated merely by increasing the dose of the wild oregano and also by taking, simultaneously, purging agents. However, regarding daily intake there are no concerns such as toxicity to the internal organs. There is no possibility of liver or kidney damage from the intake in the suggested doses of natural spice oils, particularly edible spice oils such as oil of oregano, coriander oil, oil of sage, oil of clove bud, and oil of cinnamon bark. Moreover, this is only true of those oils which are derived strictly from edible plants and also the edible part of the plant.

Some people are concerned about when the wild oregano can be taken. This is largely irrelevant. The only issue in this regard is for those with sensitive stomachs. In this case the oregano can be taken with a full meal. Otherwise, there is no difference whether it is taken morning, noon, or night. Others wonder if it is acceptable to take the oregano at night or at bedtime. In fact, this is an ideal time to take it. Much of the healing processes of the body occur at night, especially during sleep. It is of great benefit to the body to take the oregano during this time. Nor is there any concern that this would disturb sleep. On the contrary with its natural morphine-like action the oregano, especially the juice and the oil, is a natural sedative. For many people the oil and/or juice taken at bedtime acts as a highly effective sleep aid. This is particularly true of those who have great difficulty falling asleep.

Regarding the natural bacteria in the intestines the germicidal powers of wild oregano oil are a definite issue. In high doses the oregano oil can kill the healthy bacteria. This is easy to remedy. It can be done by increasing the intake of yogurt and also by taking a healthy bacterial supplement. Such a supplement should be taken at night, away from the wild oregano dosing. This can be taken merely an hour after any final oregano dose.

The whole herb complex with *Rhus coriaria* is not an issue with the healthy bacteria. In one study the whole herb actually improved the growth of these bacteria.

Too, for the gut bacteria modest doses of the oil of wild oregano are harmless such as a few drops twice daily. Anyone who must take major doses can simply take the healthy bacterial supplement and the yogurt daily or even every other day. Regardless, there is no issue of concern. The healthy bacteria readily regenerate after heavy-dose wild oregano therapy. Notably, raw garlic, too, causes the destruction of the healthy bacteria.

The oregano can be taken both with food and on an empty stomach. For people who are not used to it in general it is best to take it with food. Regarding medication, this is also largely insignificant. Wild oregano is a food or more correctly a food-spice. Thus, just as no one would wonder about the interactions of, for instance, eating nuts and seeds or eating a pizza with the wild oregano, similarly, no one should fret over taking oregano supplements with medications. The point is the oregano can do no harm. Nor does it ever cause fatality. Yet, the drugs cause great harm and vast fatality. In the United States alone it is estimated that, yearly, medications cause at a minimum some 400,000 deaths. This is based upon data published in the *Journal of the American Medical Association* (*JAMA*), where it was determined that, yearly, hundreds of thousands of people die in hospitals prematurely. All this is a result of drug therapy. Then, it is not truly a therapy but is, rather, a curse.

Worrying about the so-called toxicity or interactions of wild oregano is a waste of time or at a minimum a distraction. Regardless, the oregano oil, for instance, is only retained within the body for a relatively short period. It is quickly dissipated. Thus, it is virtually impossible for toxicity to occur. Even so, the real focus must be on the toxic and fatal effects of common medications as well as prescription drugs. In many major hospitals the number one cause for the admission of new patients is drug interactions. There are no known hospitalizations for 'oregano interactions', rather, the wild oregano prevents countless hospitalizations. Yet, do these same people who may fret about the possible toxicity of wild oregano—do they worry about the toxicity of the drugs which they take or even the aspirin or acetaminophen which they take casually? No one considers this, yet they should surely consider it as well as the intake of, for instance, alcohol, caffeine, and cold remedies, along with prescription drugs. This is because interactions with such drugs readily cause organ damage and could also prove fatal.

Regardless, it is best not to take drugs. Here, the danger is obvious, because, as has been mentioned, these agents intoxicate the tissues. Instead of such poisons people must rely on natural substances as a course of therapy. This is the consumption of whole and organic foods, along with the appropriate supplements or whole food concentrates. In addition, there must be plenty of exercise. Of note, the best exercise is brisk walking. This combination of diet, whole food supplements, and exercise is the true medicine of the future. People are turning to this type of medicine—this truly holistic approach—while rejecting drugs. This is because they are well aware of the great danger of pharmaceutical agents, while simultaneously being aware of the vast safety of natural medicine. No one wants to knowingly cause self-harm.

Even so, it must be reiterated that oil of wild oregano by itself isn't the entire answer. There must be a total body program to achieve optimal health. The spirit, too, must be healthy. True, some people don't like the mention of this subject. Yet, no one can deny its existence, this spiritual component of the human being.

It has been proven that compared to those who lack any goals people who have a purpose thrive superiorly in life. This purpose includes the belief in an afterlife or the meeting with God. People who hold to such a belief are to a degree less prone to disease than those who reject it. As well, it is critical to believe in the powers of natural medicine, that is for it to be most effective. In fact, this is true of any therapy. If a person doesn't believe in the therapy—then, it cannot be successful or its success will be impeded. Spiritually, the person must believe in the capacity to be cured.

It is better to believe in something than nothing. A person who refuses to recognize the Highest Power, the existence of which is obvious, is truly a lost soul. There is a health benefit to concentrate on and think about Him. To argue about this Being is a source of great consternation. Moreover, it is useless.

No human is all-powerful. Everyone knows that the universe is under a mighty control. When a person is asked, "Who made this vast universe and all that it contains?" There can only be one conclusion. That conclusion is almighty God. The realization of this is part of the cure. The denial of this is a major component of chronic illness. This is because the deep belief in this Being is a great source of peace. In other words, a person can find peace in the thought of almighty

God. In contrast, to reject Him is source of an internal fight. This consumes energy and thus causes sickness and disease. If a person is spiritually sick, if the heart of such a person is virtually dead, then, how can he/she be well? Again, to give thought to God and to bow to Him is part of the cure. This is because the devout worship of God creates peace—and all humans need this sensation. Rather than being about a certain ritual this is about recognizing the real power. It is about releasing the need for power and control and giving it all to 'the only One who is truly in control.' Some of the sickest people in the world are those who must control all issues. In contrast, those who trust in God give Him the control.

So, there are physical benefits in the belief in the higher power. There are also great benefits to be grateful to this power. The human benefits from feeling this gratitude. It is a source of peace. In contrast, refusing to feel this is the cause of great distress, the distress being lodged directly in the heart. The fact is the belief in God is a great source of comfort, true peace.

Anyone can realize this truth by merely looking up into the universe on a star-filled night. Could there be any other conclusion other than the fact that there really is only one God? For anyone who would consider it, obviously, it is this Being who created the vast universe. It is a universe that operates in a oneness. All that exists follows systems. There is no group of gods, who would clearly fight among each other. The oneness of God is obvious, but only people who give this deep thought realize it. Yet, it is only to the human's benefit to believe. Gratitude to God creates great peace in the heart. Through this gratitude there is happiness. This gratitude is the ultimate cure for the spiritually ill but is also a part of the cure for physical illness. Even so, this is not sufficient in most cases. In other words, to truly cure disease physical cures are also required. This book provides such cures.

Again, there is need for good food. There is also need for fresh air and exercise. The wild oregano will help immensely, however, the benefits for the body are far greater when all these elements are combined. In particular, fresh air and sunshine greatly enhance the powers of wild oregano.

How to find the best wild oregano: potency

Regarding the oregano oil there is a common question about potency. Understandably, people want to get the greatest value for their money. This brings up the issue of the active ingredient. Most commonly, this is known as carvacrol. There is a kind of "carvacrol war" occurring by various manufacturers. These are the imitation brands, which are sold by companies that fail to have their own manufacturing facilities. Such companies merely buy supposed oregano oil on the open market from manufacturers unknown.

In contrast, the company representing the original brand of wild oregano oil maintains its own factory in the Mediterranean locations. Here, the wild oregano, which is hand-picked from the mountains, is systematically extracted using steam. The resulting product has a wide range of natural active ingredients, one of which is carvacrol. This is the most well known oregano oil factory in the world, to which the village people bring their finest oregano. Carvacrol is measured and found to be from 60% to 75%. Higher levels are virtually unknown. Yet, there are companies claiming to have carvacrol levels of up to 85% or even 90% in their products? This is impossible. In fact, a number of such products, boasting carvacrol levels of 75% to 90% were tested. All such products had carvacrol levels less than 60%. Yet, if carvacrol levels are this high, that is 80% or more, this is derogatory. This is because such levels usually mean that the oregano is genetically engineered. These processes corrupt the quality of both the spice and the essential oil, rendering them inedible, rather, poisonous.

Rather than the level of one mere substance of greater importance is the fact that the oregano is wild and unprocessed. High carvacrol oregano plants are being genetically engineered, primarily by Israelis. The latter have specifically created genetically corrupted forms of oregano. This is in order to create a so-called standardized hybrid. In the process much of the oregano, now corrupt, must be treated with herbicides and pesticides, and these chemicals become incorporated into the oil. This fabricated oregano, as well as the oil derived from these fabricated plants, is being sold on the market. No wonder people who take such artificial oils suffer from complaints such as headache, stomachache, backache, palpitations, and heart pain. All such symptoms are being reported by people who take such unknown-source and/or artificially engineered forms of oregano oils.

Antiinflammatory powers of wild oregano

Wild oregano possesses significant antiinflammatory powers. These powers are virtually equal to those exhibited by antiinflammatory drugs. In one study published in *Phytotherapy Research* oregano oil proved to be actually more potent than common antiinflammatory drugs in suppressing inflammation. In an animal test the oil was, in fact, nearly two-thirds as effective in reducing pain as morphine. Researchers, based in Turkey, were led to the potential of oregano oil for halting inflammation because of practices of the villagers, since the common people use oregano oil for severe injuries such as broken bones, sprains, and bruises.

There are great benefits in using the oil of oregano for inflammation. There are no side effects such as those seen in common drugs. The latter may cause damage to the internal organs and are a primary cause of sudden intestinal or gastric bleeding. Plus, unlike most drugs oregano oil can be used both topically and internally.

Incredibly, the oregano oil is also an excellent remedy for pain. In particular, it is invaluable topically for the pain of arthritis, since, like oil of cayenne, which is also used for this purpose, it is heat-producing. Thus, it stimulates local blood flow. This increase in blood flow helps ease both pain and inflammation. For ideal results the oil can also be taken internally as drops under the tongue. The immense pain-killing powers of the oil is demonstrated by the following case history:

> Mr. M. is a 50-year-old male, who tends to be rambunctious about his work. He loves doing home chores but often goes overboard. Excited about a new wall addition he was building he was working in his typical furious method when he dropped a cement block on his foot. Screaming in pain, his wife came to see what happened and noticed that, quickly, his foot turned black and blue. She recalled that she had just got in the mail a bottle of the oil of wild oregano (Mediterranean-source, hand-picked and high mountain). She rubbed this all over the foot, which gave him major relief, and took him to the hospital.

The doctor examined the foot, ordered x-rays, and, thus, confirmed the fracture. Then, he said, "I press on your foot, and you have no pain. Normally, people would be screaming in pain with this type of injury. There is also no swelling, which is incredible. By the way, what is that pungent smell? It smells like a pizza."

The best type of oregano oil for pain and inflammation is the high or super-strength type. This may be rubbed directly on any inflamed or painful region. For swellings, too, the oil is effective. Here, it can rapidly reduce the swelling and is particularly valuable for mobilizing the swelling associated with trauma. It is also effective at easing and dissipating bruises. It is commonly noted that, after applying the oregano oil, the matter within the bruise is rapidly mobilized upward. This is because the oregano oil stimulates lymph flow, and it is through the lymph that the dead matter within the bruise is mobilized.

Lymph mobilization

The lymphatic system is a vast network of vessels and glands. The vessels begin in the feet and from here course throughout the tissues of the legs, pelvis, abdomen and chest. All internal organs are well supplied by a network of lymphatic vessels. These vessels ultimately enter various lymph nodes, which serve as a system for cleansing the lymph of any toxins. After the lymph has been cleansed it is dumped into the general circulation.

The lymph serves a number of critical functions. One such function is to mobilize excessive fluids and proteins. It is also to mobilize and eliminate waste protein. If the lymph is compromised, the waste protein and, therefore, fluid which is associated with it stagnate. Swellings may occur. This is known as lymphedema.

Lymphedema is usually manifested as a one-sided swelling. The condition can be differentiated from other causes of swelling by this one-sided nature. In contrast, regarding swelling in the legs if this is on both sides and appears equal, this is usually from heart failure. Swelling on both sides may also be the result of an imbalance in the glands, notably the thyroid and pituitary. Swollen ankles on both sides is usually a sign of weak pituitary function.

Usually, swelling in the lymphatic system is the result of infection. The most suspect culprit is worms, notably the filarial worm, which is the cause of elephantiasis. The lymphatics may be infected by other worms such as hookworm. Also, the one-sided swelling may be the result of surgery, where the drainage system is destroyed.

In the treatment of lymphedema wild oregano oil is a godsend. Using the super or high strength variety the oil should be vigorously scrubbed into the involved region using mainly upward strokes. This should be repeated until the swelling is eliminated. Also, the high strength oil should be taken internally, about 20 drops twice daily, again, until the condition is resolved. Other oils which help mobilize lymph include oil of wild rosemary, wild lavender oil, and oil of wild sage (all in an extra virgin olive oil base).

Fruit enzymes are also powerful in mobilizing lymph congestion. The most powerful fruit enzymes are bromelain and papain from pineapple and papaya respectively. These enzymes act virtually as chemical roto-rooter-like agents, attacking any swelling or blockage.

This supplement is available as either capsules or pressed pills. The pressed pills are rather impotent. Apparently, the process of pressing creates sufficient heat, which disables the enzymes. Capsules are the best form. Moreover, much of the papain on the market is derived from Hawaiian papaya, which is genetically engineered. Thus, the ideal supplement is from non-Hawaiian sources such as Thailand. Look for a high potency enzyme cleansing supplement, which is labeled GMO-free and which is a combination of bromelain and papain plus spice extracts, including rosemary and turmeric. For lymphatic swelling the ideal method of intake is on an empty stomach, one to three capsules three times daily. The repeated dose helps keep the blood levels of the enzymes sufficiently high, so they can do their work of decongesting the site of swelling. This enzyme therapy is particularly effective in the case of surgically-induced lymphatic swelling.

Such enzyme therapy is also effective for swellings caused by injury or infection. In fact, trauma also causes congestion of the lymphatic system. For instance, a bruise is essentially lymphatic congestion, as is the swelling of a localized bacterial infection. Thus, the protocol for the elimination of swelling caused by lymphatic congestion/injury is to rub the super/high-strength oil of wild oregano on or about the site of injury in an upward stroking fashion, to take the oil internally, ideally as sublingual drops, and to take the bromelain/papain plus wild rosemary and ginger extract high dose capsules as repeated doses. Other optional natural medicines for use in the mobilization of lymph are oils of wild rosemary, lavender, and sage, which can be added to the protocol in extreme cases. In particular, oil of wild rosemary in a base of extra virgin olive oil is highly effective in lymph mobilization.

Supplements to use along with wild oregano

The best supplements to use with wild oregano are various whole food supplements, along with wild extracts. The whole food supplements provide natural vitamins and minerals desperately needed by the body. The wild extracts, particularly wild extracts of berries and greens, help cleanse the body of toxins, which greatly assists the powers of wild oregano.

Vitamins are required for the function of all cells. The oregano therapy is most effective when taken with natural vitamin concentrates. The key natural vitamins needed to work with the oregano are vitamin C, vitamin E, vitamins A and D, and the B complex vitamins.

Natural B complex is found in a supplement made from crude rice polish, rice bran, crushed flax, and red sour grape. The ideal vitamin C is purely from natural sources, notably wild camu camu plus acerola. Regarding vitamin E virtually all the supplements on the market are derived from genetically engineered soy. The exception is a supplement derived from a non-genetically engineered source. This is sunflower seed, a source which contains the entire complex of vitamin E molecules. Check health food stores for a sunflower seed oil-derived vitamin E complex in a base of crude whole pumpkinseed oil and wild red palm oil.

The best source of vitamins A and D is salmon oil. In particular, this is the oil derived from wild Alaskan sockeye salmon. Regarding this source it is non-genetically engineered, plus it is free of heavy refinement. Unlike commercial fish oils the wild sockeye salmon oil concentrate is never treated with harsh chemicals. While detergents and deodorants are used in the processing of standard fish oil supplements no such chemicals are used in the processing of the polar-source sockeye salmon oil. It is extracted using only steam. It undergoes no other treatment. The crude rice polish/bran supplement provides much of the B complex. In particular, it provides thiamine and niacin in rich amounts plus a good amount of pyridoxine and biotin. However, there is no B_{12} in such a supplement. The content of riboflavin is also minimal. To procure B_{12} it is necessary to eat red meat and egg yolk. However, liver is the top source of this nutrient. The occasional consumption of organic liver from cows, calves, and/or lamb amply supplies this nutrient.

For riboflavin organic whole milk, or, preferably, raw milk, is the best source, although liver is even more dense in this nutrient. Other top sources are egg yolk, cheese, and dark green leafy vegetables. Regarding a supplemental source wild greens drops derived from raw extracts of dandelion, burdock, and nettle leaves, are supremely rich. A mere ounce of such drops contains about one milligram of this key vitamin, which is considerable. Thus, these drops serve as a riboflavin supplement. Again, the active ingredients are mainly derived from wild raw greens, that is nettles, burdock, and dandelion. These are remote-source greens, which are free of pollution. These wild greens have a dramatic action on the liver, greatly increasing bile production.

A side effect of taking these greens is an obvious improvement of bowel function. This type of cleansing, this wild greens purging, is necessary to prevent the intestinal tract from degenerating. Sluggish intestinal function leads to inflammation of the intestinal walls, which then may lead to a variety of diseases, including arthritis, Crohn's disease, ulcerative colitis, spastic colon, fibromyalgia, gastritis, migraine headaches, esophageal reflux, skin inflammation, and cancer. All this is prevented by the regular intake of a crude raw wild greens complex, as drops under the tongue).

Thus, for optimal health of the immune system, as well as all other body systems, the following nutritional supplements should ideally be taken, along with the wild oregano:

- a crude whole rice polish/bran concentrate, combined with crushed whole fortified flax and red sour grape
- a northern polar-source Alaskan sockeye salmon fish oil, extracted only with steam, nutrients intact, as a key source of vitamins A and, particulary, vitamin D
- a wild camu camu and acerola-based natural vitamin C complex
- a sunflower seed oil-source natural vitamin E complex (non-GMO, soy-free)
- organic liver or egg yolks as a B_{12} source
- a wild raw greens complex as a riboflavin source
- raw whole organic milk as a source of vitamin D and riboflavin
- raw Andes-source purple maca drops as a source of vegetable-source vitamin B_{12} as well as vitamin D
- a wild raw eight berries complex as drops under-the-tongue (as a source of polyphenols)

Consider this list. Obviously, it is food and its extracts that are the true cures. In contrast, chemical-based vitamins have no place in this program. Natural nutrients are far safer than the chemical types plus they are more effective in both the reversal of disease and the maintenance of ideal health. These completely natural nutrients, as found in whole foods, are critical for cellular functions. The cells thrive on these nutrients; the body readily absorbs all such nutrients from the food supplements. In contrast, the body rejects synthetic nutrients, dumping them through the stool and into the urine.

As a result of the deficiency of key nutrients great imbalances occur in the body. This leads to a decline in overall health. A lack of B vitamins impairs the production of energy in the body. Also, the synthesis of neurotransmitters in the nervous system is disrupted. In addition, the synthesis of protein is largely dependent upon these nutrients.

Vitamin C is essential for the maintenance of the skeletal system. The vitamin is essential for the strengthening of the walls of veins and arteries. It is greatly needed by the glands, particularly the pituitary and adrenal glands. Regarding the latter the synthesis of adrenal steroids is dependent upon adequate levels of vitamin C. Then, it is the adrenal glands which largely control the germ killing power of the immune system. People with adrenal exhaustion invariably suffer from a severe vulnerability to infection. To some degree adrenal exhaustion is due to vitamin C deficiency. That is how important is this nutrient to adrenal function—because, without it, there is no way to adequately produce the adrenal steroids. The best way to infuse the adrenal glands with vitamin C is to consume the crude whole food sources.

Vitamin E is required for healthy circulation. It is also a key antioxidant. To keep the immune and circulatory systems in balance it is necessary to take this nutrient on a daily basis. The best supplemental sources of this vitamin are the following:

- sunflower seed oil vitamin E, as capsules or sublingual drops, combined with crude extracts of pumpkinseed and red palm oil
- crude whole cold-pressed Austrian pumpkinseed oil
- crude whole cold-pressed wild-source red palm oil
- crude Turkish-source cold-pressed sesame oil

Vitamins A and D are also key components for a healthy body. The oregano therapy is most optimal when these nutrients are in a rich supply. Both these nutrients are required for the strength of the skeleton. Vitamin A is essential for the health/strength of the various cell linings of the body. These linings are made of epithelial cells. The synthesis of these critical cells is dependent upon vitamin A. This function of vitamin A is of the utmost importance. The cell linings of the various organs are the body's first line of defense. To ward off disease these linings must be in ideal condition. Without vitamin A the linings degenerate. This allows the establishment of disease and, possibly, the growth of cancer. Regardless, it is important to consume the vitamin A through unprocessed natural sources. Only this type of vitamin A is effective in preventing the deficiency and, as well, healing deficiency-damaged tissues.

Vitamin D serves a similar function for the bones and joints. Here, it is responsible for mineral deposition, particularly the deposition of calcium and phosphorus. A strong skeleton is also a defense against disease. This vitamin is also involved in the growth of cells, for instance, in the prostate. Without it, prostate cells grow recklessly, which may lead to cancer. The same is true of vitamin A, because in a deficiency there can be significant overgrowth of the cells which line the internal organs such as the cells which line the mouth, intestines, and lungs. In vitamin C deficiency the linings of the tissues are also negatively affected, in fact, they degenerate. So, it becomes obvious how such nutrients work in unison with the wild oregano—to balance the immune system and to, ultimately, prevent and cure disease. Again, all these vitamins can be consumed through natural whole foods as well as whole food supplements.

This was the original method of vitamin therapy, that is the method used before the chemical synthesis of these compounds. Originally, doctors such as D. C. Munro, author of *Man Alive*, used only natural concentrates in the treatment of deficiency diseases. Yet, incredibly, such early practitioners, real experts in natural medicine, such as Drs. Munro, McCarrison, and Price, also used these concentrates for the treatment of serious diseases. In contrast, none of these great men, true pioneers in their fields, used chemical vitamins. Rather, they proved that symptoms and diseases were readily reversed through the use of foods packing high concentration of the key nutrients.

The main concentrates which were used included fish liver oils, rice bran concentrates, B vitamin-rich yeasts, liver, egg yolk, lemon juice, and similar whole food sources. After the discovery of vitamins this was what was originally used in the cure of disease. The chemical vitamins came later and have, in contrast, never been shown to be curative. This is why in this book only food sources of nutrients are recommended. For reasons that defy scientists the natural or food sources of vitamins and minerals help heal the body, while the synthetic or man-made types never achieve this.

The same is true of flavonoids. Only the natural, whole, crude sources offer the potency to heal and cure. This was determined by Stoner and his group at Ohio State University, when he studied flavonoid-rich berries. Here, it was determined that the whole unprocessed berry, in this instance black raspberries, alone was curative, while extracts of supposed active ingredients were only modestly effective. Thus, regarding the ultimate effects in the body the synthetic and natural are not the same, but, rather, there is a vast difference, with the natural type being the only kind which induces physiological changes. Nor are man-made extracts, where the whole food is fragmented, as powerful as the complete whole substance. This proves that human intelligence is limited and that the real intelligence derives from the creator, who knows the inner workings of all that is. This is what is repeatedly found. For vitamins, minerals, flavonoids, enzymes, phenolic compounds, and polyphenols it is only the truly natural whole food sources which are effective in the treatment and reversal of disease. It is also only these which are entirely safe for human consumption, even in relatively large amounts.

Of note, it is important to reiterate that virtually all the studies done showing a positive effect of food and nutrients on disease are based on only food or food sources. In contrast, when studies are done using synthetic vitamins, the results are poor. There are studies which demonstrate that there is no obvious effect from such man-made vitamins. In some instances the synthetic vitamins have even been found to worsen the conditions. Thus, truly natural substances, the medicines of the almighty creator, are the only hope for cure for the countless diseases, which afflict humankind. No chemical produced in a lab, including synthetic vitamins and minerals, is effective. In contrast, the lycopene of tomatoes, the essential oil of oregano, the B vitamins of rice bran, the vitamin D of fish oil, the vitamin C of acerola, camu camu, and lemon juice are all effective in the reversal of serious symptoms and life threatening diseases.

It is worth reiterating. Food itself is curative, for instance, the studies of Gary Stoner and his group at Ohio State University on berries. Here, Stoner found that freeze dried berries, notably black raspberries, are more effective than any known drug in the destruction of tumors. Furthermore, raw honey has been determined as curative, studies showing that it halts diarrhea, as well as irritating coughs, and does so better than any drug. Regarding oil of oregano a preliminary study showed that this powerful substance effectively reversed hepatitis C in six patients, proving more effective than the standard drug for this disease. So, for the vast ailments of humankind there is great hope. But rather than in the realm of the scientist or chemist this will be found in the elements of nature, which are the unaltered and pure whole foods and their concentrates. These are the original cures, which have been used since the beginning of humankind.

There are powerful forces which are attempting to prevent people from using the powers of nature. These forces are attempting to interfere with peoples' rights to choose completely natural medicines or, rather, supplements purely for selfish purposes. These are the pharmaceutical houses, supported by the chemical-industrial complex. Then, the great power behind this is the industrial petrochemical cartel, which includes the oil barons. It is these powerful ones who are largely responsible for the repression of natural medicine, all as a means to maintain the sales of chemical drugs.

People should resist this by refusing to use their wares. It is necessary to boycott all drugs, because the drug companies are plotting against the people. Those who take drugs do poorly and live a shorter life versus those who never take them. What's more, the number one cause of fatality in the United States is no longer heart disease but, rather, it is drug toxicity. In many hospitals the main cause for sudden critical admission of patients is drug reaction. The primary cause of complaint to the FDA by parents, that is regarding sudden and potentially fatal illnesses in children or even fatality, is vaccine reaction. In contrast, there are no complaints by parents or people in general to the government of disease/sickness from, for instance, spice-based oil of wild oregano, tomato-source lycopene, raw wild honey, wild raw berry extracts, or wild raw greens extracts. So, why is the government attempting to regulate and weaken the nutritional supplement industry? It is only because the pharmaceutical and oil industries *are* the government. In other words, the government has been created to serve certain industries and the powerful people, which represent them.

People have influence through their purchasing power. If people refuse to support such tyranny, then, there can be impact. Thus, for those who seek freedom of choice and who seek the unbiased truth buying any kind of pharmaceutical drug, even minor over-the-counter types, is destructive. It is destructive because by purchasing these drugs they are supporting precisely the powers which seek to weaken them, to diminish their opportunities, and to essentially steal their freedoms. Thus, concerned and dedicated people must boycott the drug companies. These companies are doing nothing productive for the human race. Their claims are purely bogus.

Anyone who wishes to confirm this can read the book by the former editor-in-chief of the *New England Journal of Medicine*, Marsha Angell, M.D. This book, *The Truth About the Drug Companies*, tells the inside truth of the fraud and corruption of the drug cartel. Angell exposes how the people behind this so-called industry purposely deceive people to sell them their wares, even if it means putting their lives at risk. She states the situation very simply. The drug companies, she says, operate by deceit. In other words, like the tobacco companies, these companies make it their intention to sell their wares at all costs, even the cost of human lives. They convince the people of the validity through mere corruption. This is, Angell makes clear, through fabricating their research. This is to gain a false sense of trust from the people. The drug companies bribe people, she says, to fake their way into the market. Virtually none of the modern drugs, she notes, are based upon any sound science. This means their claims are bogus. Rather, the drugs which they produce are sold solely on marketing pitches—and there is no sound basis for their use. Even so, people have been convinced by marketing to take them. Angell makes it clear—and as a nearly 20 year veteran as the Editor-in-Chief of the prestigious *New England Journal of Medicine* she is a certain authority—that contrary to claims today's pharmaceutical drugs are not only unproven but they also are unsafe.

The fact that the science is fabricated is sufficient reason to ban these drugs. Regardless, why anyone would support such groups by buying their drugs is unfathomable. Every penny which is spent for the drug companies results in some degree of oppression. This is through funding a system based upon lies. If it is fear of death which is the cause of this support. If this is why people clamor to take their products, then, this is even more bizarre, since by trusting in pharmaceutical products and by taking these preparations the opposite occurs: the incidence of death rises dramatically. Again, people who take no drugs live significantly longer than those who take them. Also, people who take exclusively natural cures never die from sudden death because of such cures, while for those who take drugs sudden death is a relatively common occurrence.

Chapter Nine

Oregano and Athletics

For athletes and sports enthusiasts wild oregano is a boon. This is especially true of the steam distilled oil. This oil has immense value for muscular injuries as well as injuries to joints and bones. For cuts and open wounds of all types it is unsurpassed. It is also invaluable for burns and scrapes. In fact, for any sudden injury to the body wild oregano finds significant use. Oregano has a number of properties which makes it ideal for athletics. It has much trapped energy, which, when consumed through eating the wild crude herb or taking the extracts, is released into the body. This energy increases the rate of metabolism. In other words, through the intake of wild oregano there is an increase in energy production. Also, wild oregano is naturally rich in oxygen. This is particularly true of the steam extracted essence or juice. This oxygen is of great utility in muscle cell metabolism. For athletes this means an increase in the degree of muscular strength as well as stamina.

Additionally, oregano is a potent antioxidant. This means that it is a cellular preservative. As an antioxidant the oregano helps prevent toxic damage to the cells, the damage that typically occurs from overuse of the body. Here, heavy athletic activity causes an increase in oxidative stress to the tissues, which oregano largely blocks. Moreover, oregano is a water-phase antioxidant. This means it is highly active in the blood and within the cell substance. For athletes who are involved in competitive sports this is the ideal type of antioxidant to consume. The muscles are mostly water weight. Thus, a water-phase antioxidant, such as the wild oregano, will readily penetrate these tissues, helping prevent or reverse oxidative damage. The same is true of the oregano essence or juice. It is the oxidative damage secondary to muscular activity, which has everything to do with the degree of stamina and power exhibited by athletes. So, of all antioxidants for increasing the effectiveness of athletic performance wild oregano is supreme. The best forms of wild oregano to use are the steam distilled oil, the crude whole herb with *Rhus coriaria*, and the steam distilled essence or juice.

Scientific studies give evidence of this power. A study was done on the muscles of animals, that is rabbits, to determine how oregano would modify oxidative stress, the same stress which occurs due to exercise. Control rabbits were fed the regular diet, while the contrary group was fed this diet plus oil of oregano in considerable amounts, some 100 to 200 milligrams per kilogram of food. In the oregano oil-fed group it was found that the level of oxidative damage to muscular tissue was much lower than in controls. The conclusion is that regular consumption of oregano oil exerts a 'significant antioxidant effect,' with the higher intake being most effective. This means that, when the muscles are stressed, oregano oil prevents damage to the muscle lipids, that is the fatty cell wall components of muscle cells. The substance measured for determining oxidative damage of muscle cells is malondialdehyde, and this substance was elevated in the rabbits given no oregano and much reduced in those given large amounts of the oil. This is a significant result. It means that the oregano oil helps reverse any exercise-induced damage to the tissues. In addition, vitamin E was found to be effective in reducing body levels of this compound. Thus, for ideal results in boosting athletic performance the oregano oil should be consumed, along with a natural source vitamin E such as the non-genetically engineered sunflower seed-source vitamin E in a crude cold-pressed pumpkinseed oil base. Vitamin E proved in this study to be slightly more powerful than oregano oil in reducing muscle-stress oxidative damage. The consumption of these two antioxidants together is a highly potent means to prevent exercise-induced oxidative damage. Thus, the athletic individual should consider the daily intake of oil of wild oregano (Mediterranean-source), juice of wild oregano, and sunflower seed oil-source vitamin E.

Again, for vitamin E be sure to use only non-GM sources. This rules out all soy oil-based vitamin E. Only vitamin E from sunflower seed oil, red palm oil, rice bran oil, and/or wheat germ oil is free of GMOs. The genetically modified type of vitamin E has been associated with an increased risk for sudden death due to heart disorders, whereas, in contrast, GMO-free sources of vitamin E protect the body from heart attacks. Genetic engineering concentrates toxins in the final product. Athletes should avoid all sources of genetically engineered vitamin E.

It is well known that wild oregano creates power. This power is because of its potent action upon the immune system as well as its antioxidant action. It is also because it is a sun-charged plant, and when ingested, these energy charges are released into the body. It is the antioxidant action which is critical for preserving cell function, and, surely, the cells are stressed from aggressive exercise.

There is yet another key action for which oregano is responsible. This relates to its action on the heart muscle. Oregano is a strengthener of muscle tissue, and the heart is no exception. According to Turkish investigators wild oregano is a positive ionotrope. An ionotrope is a substance which has direct actions upon the heart muscle, that is by effecting the heart's muscle contractions. A positive ionotrope is a substance which boosts the heart contractions, essentially strengthening its pumping actions. In contrast, a negative ionotrope interferes with the contractions, weakening the pumping power.

Of all types of wild oregano extracts it is the juice or essence which exerts the most powerful 'positive' actions on the heart muscle. Noted the Turkish researchers this juice has a significant action on the heart muscle, increasing its strength comparable to any drug.

There is also the issue of wild oregano's antiinflammatory as well as anti-pain actions. It was, again, Turkish investigators who first revealed this. The revelation was based upon folk use of the oil, since for Turkish villagers it is a common remedy for arthritis as well as trauma. Using an animal model the investigators discovered a surprising finding. When compared to common antiinflammatory agents, such as the so-called non-steroidal antiinflammatory agents, for the reduction of pain oregano oil was superior to such drugs. In fact, the oregano oil proved so powerful in this preliminary study that it was nearly two-thirds as effective as morphine.

Athletes are plagued with fungal infections. Some athletes suffer from massive fungal overload, both internally and externally. Here, the oregano oil is a boon. It obliterates fungi, whether on or in the body. For deep-seated fungal infections, however, patience is necessary. It may take a few months to truly cleanse the body of such fungal invasion. Yet, eventually, the wild oregano will purge the fungus, and all will be well. To accelerate this purge it is also useful to take a high quality natural bacterial supplement. Regardless, such fungal infections are an impediment to ideal athletic performance. This is particularly true of internal infestation, which disrupts energy production but also causes inflammation. Even so, any external infestation is a sign that, internally, there is also significant infection.

There is also evidence that the wild oregano helps in tissue growth. This may be a function of its power in boosting digestion. The wild oregano has a powerful effect on stomach function as well as the function of the upper small intestine, increasing the flow of digestive secretions. It is also a modest anti-hyperglycemic agent, that is it acts to preserve the function of the pancreas. Thus, for muscle building the wild oregano should be added to the menu as the crude whole herb sprinkled on food in relatively large quantities such as a tablespoon or more twice daily.

So, wild oregano is, perhaps, the athlete's most versatile natural medicine. It possesses antioxidant, antiinflammatory, anti-pain, anti-swelling, anti-bruising, wound healing, energizing, and heart strengthening powers. Plus, it alone has the massive power of cleansing the tissues of both internal and external fungal infections. Furthermore, a wild oregano-based emulsified spray can be used to decontaminate athletic environments therefore preventing outbreaks of destructive and even deadly germs.

Athletes are highly vulnerable to infections. This is particularly true of those who travel extensively by airplane, especially during the winter. The wild oregano is exceedingly protective here and if taken regularly will largely prevent the occurrence of common infections such as colds, flu, sore throat, laryngitis, and tonsillitis. Thus, the wild oregano in the form of the steam distilled oil, the crude whole herb plus *Rhus coriaria*, and the juice could be that secret substance that makes the difference between mediocrity and greatness in the athletic field. In this regard it is one of the secrets of certain professional teams which have benefited significantly since using wild oregano-based supplements.

How to use wild oregano in athletes

The best form of oregano to take for strength is the whole crude herb, along with the juice. The crude herb can be taken as a daily supplement. The juice may be drunk immediately before a performance or in the midst of it. A shot of the juice can be taken for the generation of great power. Moreover, this can be used repeatedly. This juice will create both energy and courage, the later being highly necessary in many sports. For injuries and wounds the oil is the most effective. Here, it can be rubbed topically repeatedly and also can be taken internally. It is ideal for sprains, strains, pulled muscles, ligamentous injuries, contusions, abrasions, and cuts. In addition, regarding fractures wild oregano speeds the healing, and the best types to consume are the crude herb and the oil.

The crude herb helps increase bone density, and therefore, speeds the healing of any skeletal injury. The spray can be used to liven the senses and to activate the brain centers. It can also be used to decontaminate athletic surfaces and body parts to prevent the onset or spread of infection. It is effective against athletes foot. As well, the cream, based upon a 6%

solution of essential oils in a base of raw honey, Canada balsam, and propolis, can be used to heal open or raw wounds as well as abrasions and burns. Other supplements useful in athletics are the whole food wild-source vitamin C, both as capsules and drops under the tongue. The drops under the tongue, made from wild-source camu camu, passion fruit, and palm fruits, creates great energy—and this is quick energy, which is immediately noticeable. There is also the raw maca drops with purple corn, which also gives immense energy. Since these drops are rich in hormones this is also a source for power, that is in those sports where this is desired. In addition, there is the natural-source vitamin E from sunflower seed oil. Such vitamin E helps oxygenate the blood, and the benefits of this in athletics are obvious.

For athletes and more: home uses of wild oregano

There are countless uses for wild oregano in the home. The benefits of relying upon such a broad spectrum antiseptic are obvious. Wild oil of oregano can be added to virtually all home solutions to increase antiseptic powers as well as, incredibly, cleaning capacity. Wild oregano has solvent properties, and, thus, it assists in the cleaning process. In addition, the antiseptic spray containing various spice oils is a powerful cleaner as well as spot remover. The oil may be added to the wash cycle to sterilize and freshen clothes. The same is true of the spray, which can be misted into the washing, as well as drying, cycle.

The crude herb makes a fine food additive. It may be added to any soup, salad dressing, or dip. It may also be sprinkled on meat and fish dishes. There is no damage to such oregano supplements through cooking.

For pump soaps and shampoos wild oregano oil makes an ideal additive. This will help keep hands, body, and scalp free of infections. Of note, infections of the scalp are exceedingly common. Moreover, balding has recently been associated with infection of the scalp with not only fungi but also hair follicle mites. The mites actually thrive in the follicles and eat the hair roots, causing hair loss, including male pattern baldness. These mites are thoroughly destroyed by wild oregano.

For pests the multiple spice spray is ideal. Regarding ants this will usually either kill them or drive them away. For mosquitos it makes an effective repellent. Sprayed on screens it helps keep them away. It may also be misted about in the air at picnics and other outings to prevent mosquito attacks. A great benefit here is that this spray is safe for misting about food and beverages. It is also safe for use on infants, babies, and toddlers.

The cleaning and deodorizing powers of both oregano oil and, particularly, the oregano oil-based multiple spice spray are remarkable. Cleaning, protection, and deodorization can be achieved anywhere on the body. For instance, the oil or spray put into shampoo eliminates hair odors. Sprayed on the body offensive odors are eliminated. The spray makes the ideal underarm deodorant as well as sanitizer. Misted on the body the entire body tissues are vitalized. For odors in the genital region one or two mists from a distance of a foot or two is sufficient. This would aid in the prevention of urinary and/or vaginal infections.

For the feet both the oil and spray mist are ideal. The oil may be rubbed on the bottom of the feet daily, a few drops rubbed into each foot. For foot odors also the spray is highly effective. The same is true of bothersome athlete's foot fungus, as both the spray and oil are highly active against foot fungi. As well, for deodorizing shoes there is no product as effective as the multiple spice spray. This spray is also effective for cleaning mud from shoes and for sterilizing them. The inner linings of tennis shoes in particular are readily infected by fungi. Regular misting with the multiple spice spray prevents this.

Chapter Ten

Mutant Germs: Modern Plague

The fight against mutant germs isn't lost. This is because these germs are readily destroyed by spice oils. Repeatedly, in all tests performed these germs succumb when exposed to these oils. The most powerful of these is the oil of wild oregano. This is perhaps the ultimate proof of the power of wild oregano oil. Mutant germs are a vast cause of human disability. The germs routinely maim individuals. Consider the so-called flesh eating bacteria, which can rapidly destroy human flesh. More ominously, yearly, all over the globe such germs cause countless deaths. In the United States alone every year some 300,000 people die from infections caused by mutants.

The mutants are a medical disaster, that is they are the consequence of modern medicine. They are the side effect of the excessive use of antibiotics. For years medical experts have warned of the impending crisis but to no avail. Even Alexander Fleming, discoverer of penicillin, gave due warning. Even during his lifetime he saw the development of resistant germs and warned that unless antibiotics were used judiciously, ultimately, their usefulness would decline and drug-resistant germs would become a plague. His words are prophetic, yet since his time thousands of other experts have issued similar warnings. Doctors refuse to heed these warnings and continue to over-prescribe these drugs, resulting in the creation of highly dangerous mutants. Then, these noxious germs, which are no longer vulnerable to antibiotics, cause infections, which are often devastating. Much of this devastation could be prevented if only the doctors would prescribe the wild oregano oil. This is because this oil obliterates the mutants with very few if any exceptions.

In a high quality animal study at Georgetown University the wild high mountain oregano proved effective in killing drug resistant mutants. This is an incredible feat; a natural product comes to the rescue against a man-made, rather, pharmaceutical-induced catastrophe. In the entire pharmaceutical world not a single cure for this crisis has been created. Here, the pharmaceutical cartel has failed miserably. The cartel has not only created the disaster but has also proved incompetent to solve it. Yet, indisputably, the oregano oil proved at a minimum equal to the most powerful drug, Vancomycin, used to treat drug resistant infections. In this study mice were infected with penicillin-resistant staph. The control mice, given only olive oil, all died, while half the drug-treated and oregano-treated mice survived. Yet, the researchers concluded that the oregano oil proved superior, since it was less harsh than the antibiotics on the test animals than the drug.

Other studies have shown the oregano's power. According to a study sponsored by the FDA oregano oil proved capable of obliterating drug-resistant E. coli. European investigators also destroyed this bacteria with the oil. As mentioned previously a preliminary study by R. Mitchell showed that the most deadly of all infections, MRSA, that is methicillin resistant *Staphylococcus aureus* (MRSA), was defeated. In this study the germ was plated on petri dishes and then the oregano oil, as the super-strength form, was added. Some 90% of all bacteria were destroyed. The spray form of the wild oregano oil, which contains not only oregano oil but also oils of cumin, cinnamon and clove, was even more effective than the oregano oil. When sprayed into the petri dish, virtually all the bacteria, amounting to tens of millions of germs, were destroyed. This is surely proof of the lifesaving powers of this potent natural extract. Yet, incredibly, the powerful ones in Western governments show no interest in taking advantage of this, of spreading this information among the people. This is despite the fact that lives are being senselessly lost because of drug resistant infections, which could be cured using the oil of oregano. The best supplements for MRSA are the super-strength oil of wild oregano, the multiple spice spray, and the multiple spice capsules.

This is not to claim any cure. Even so, there is good data demonstrating the powers of such extracts. Yet, even so, there are those who claim that "Oregano oil is unproven." Attempts are made to sanction those who proclaim its value, even though it is based upon sound science. Even with these achievements, even with the obvious interest of the U.S. government in spice oils, the latter being an obvious proof of its powers, since the government is run by big business it is no surprise that oregano oil is attacked. Yet, despite all the studies which have been done at the government level there is still the demand for ever-more science. However, incredibly, while any detractors are making such claims for the need of "more proof" countless millions of people are becoming sickened or are dying senselessly. It is senseless because these lives would be saved through wild oregano therapy. Regardless, the human race has held the wild oregano in the highest esteem over the centuries, frequently proclaiming this as a most potent natural cure. No matter, whatever the U.S. government dictates this is supposedly law. It must be the truth. No one can defy it without risk of sanction or even imprisonment. This is despite the fact that this is mentioned in scripture, in the Bible, as the most powerful natural medicine known.

Can anyone imagine it? People are imprisoned for saving lives and for helping prevent human despair. Again, imprisonment and being sanctioned is the cost for saving human lives? This is the degree to which humanity has descended. The powerful ones who control the government perpetrate these acts against their fellow humans. They do so merely for financial gain but also for control. What a shame, because all such people, too, would benefit from using the natural cures. Despite this, every effort is made to fight anyone who brings forth the cure(s), which are safe, non-toxic, and relatively inexpensive, that is compared to high-powered treatments and procedures such as by-pass surgery, chemotherapy, and radiation therapy. Anyone who attempts to help all humanity through natural, safe medicines is haughtily resisted. Since modern times the natural medicine movement has always been fought, usually successfully to the degree that the pharmaceutical cartel maintains its monopoly. Yet, this monopoly is maintained at a monumental cost. It is the cost of countless human lives.

There are people who have no real faith in natural medicine. They believe all that the doctors say, treating them as if they are virtual divinities. Whatever the doctor says must be true, is the attitude, and, thus, people submit to any dictate. Surely, they have a right to do so, as this is a world of free choice. Yet, the statistics are impossible to deny. This is because those who regularly take medication fare considerably more poorly than those who never take it. There is a well known statistic, which supports this. In the late 1970s when physicians went on strike in New York State it only took six months for people to start living longer. In other words, statistically, when doctors were unable to treat people with their caustic medical therapies—toxic drugs and dangerous surgeries—there was a significant increase in lifespan.

So, why would anyone submit to the medical approach, knowing full well that rather than saving lives it increases the death rate? With rare exceptions, such as surgical emergencies or the removal of obstructive cancerous tumors, it is better to do nothing rather than to submit to this system. There are far too many unnecessary surgeries and drugs which are administered, with the consequence of serious side effects and even fatality. Yet, all such side effects and fatalities are preventable. Again, dangerous medical procedures and potentially poisonous drugs should only be used in life-threatening circumstances. The needless ruination of lives should be banned. The great God made all people sanctified. To senselessly take a life is a crime, as is the wanton maiming and disfiguring of people, again, all for the sake of profits and power.

Oregano is the answer—the right oregano

When buying oregano oil, the quality is the issue. Not all oregano oil is the same. The same is true of the whole crude herb. There must be a degree of investigation to be sure it is the truly wild oregano. Farm-raised is inappropriate and may prove toxic. With farm-raised types there is usually the use of pesticides and herbicides, which are, then, concentrated into the final product. In addition, the oregano oil or herb may not even be true oregano oil, being derived, instead, from various oregano-like and non-oregano species. This includes the so-called Spanish thyme. The oil from this plant has a tinny taste, a kind of bitterness. It is not only inedible but is also to a degree poisonous. Oils derived from Mexican oregano are also poisonous, as the Mexican plant is not a true oregano but is, rather, a type of sage. Rather, it is a kind of sage-brush, which merely smells like oregano.

The real oregano is Mediterranean from the Fertile Crescent. This is the truly wild type of oregano, which is the food spice. This type of oregano grows wild in the highest parts of the deep Mediterranean mountains in regions such as Turkey, Greece, and Syria. This is the original site of true wild oregano species, the same type mentioned biblically. Look for guaranteed wild oregano supplements which are from hand-picked high mountain oregano. This is the actual spice oregano, which is the most powerful, as well as safe, type. Such wild oregano may be found as the oil, the whole crushed herb, and the essence or juice. It is also the type found in the cream and spray. All such forms are effective in the battle against drug resistant germs.

As mentioned previously there are derivatives of the oil, including the spray. This spray is highly effective against drug resistant germs and can kill these germs on contact as well as on surfaces and in the air.

Moreover, germs are, globally, the major cause of sudden death. They are also the key cause of chronic illness. So, the immense value of a natural broad-spectrum germicide becomes obvious. This is precisely the function of the oil of wild oregano. Its killing capacity tells of its powers, since it destroys all categories of germs—viruses, bacteria, fungi, molds, mites, and parasites. There is no other substance, synthetic or natural, which does this. This is why it is invaluable to the human race. This is also why it is capable of routinely saving lives. Again, globally, germs continuously cause deaths. If these germs can be safely killed, then, lives will be saved. No doubt, the use of wild oregano and other spice products is preserving life. For instance, through the wild oregano therapy people are being rescued from the consequences of flu as well as pneumonia, which is sudden death. There is also rescue from the consequences of diarrhea, another major killer, since the wild oregano halts this. Diarrhea can be fatal, largely because of dehydration and the loss of electrolytes. By killing the causative germ(s) the oregano eliminates the danger. Strep and staph can prove fatal and are the cause of flesh eating bacterial infections. Strep can also cause severe kidney damage and even kidney failure. Again, the wild oregano, in the form of the oil, ideally the high strength form, prevents these consequences.

Then, there are the chronic infections, which cause great disability and which may, ultimately, lead to premature death. These are the infections which smolder in the body and which no one can readily diagnose. In other words, no medical person can "prove" that these infections exist through culturing the germ. Even so, in modern medicine it is admitted that infections are the key cause of chronic conditions. For instance, consider stomach and esophageal disorders. Hiatus hernia, chronic heartburn, gastritis, and esophagitis are all caused by infections. Even esophageal and gastric (stomach) cancer are all admittedly caused by bacterial infection, that is infection by H. pylori. In addition, there may be infections by yeasts and molds. Medical journals relate that 80% of the cases of arthritis are caused by infection and that in some cases, for instance, in children diabetes is due to infection. It is also now known that a minimum of one-third of all cancers are infection-induced. This is just what is known by the orthodox medical profession. Earlier investigators, including 19th century British and Irish physicians, regarded the relationship far higher, attributed nearly all cancers to infection (see the *Cause for Cancer Revealed*, same author, Knowledge House Publishers). Here, it has been determined, vaccination causes cancer by introducing bizarre and mutated germs, which infect the immune system, destabilizing it.

The pediatrician Mendelson, author of *Confessions of a Medical Heretic,* revealed that in his practice virtually all the leukemia cases were vaccine-induced. In my own experience through taking careful histories a similar trend becomes obvious. Virtually all the children and teenagers I have evaluated with leukemia have been heavily vaccinated, and the vaccines played a clear role in the decline of their health. The same is true of individuals with lymphoma, both teenagers and adults. There is no doubt about it those who are vaccinated suffer from a decline in overall health, while those who never receive these shots enjoy more robust health.

Vaccines introduce a wide range of pathogens, which become established in the tissues. The wild oregano/multiple spice therapy clears such pathogens from the tissues. This leads to a regeneration in health. The pathogens suppress the immune system and thus it is unable to purge them from the body. Thus, through aggressive use of spice extracts there is major prevention for the human being by clearing various pathogens from the body. According to the Bible the best natural medicine for achieving this is wild oregano, known as the "hyssop of the law." The Jewish physician of the Islamic

Empire, Maimonides (12th century) stated categorically that the hyssop of the law is the wild oregano which grows in the mountains and which the villagers use on food. This is precisely the oregano used by the original makers of wild oregano supplements, the high quality brand(s) found in better health food stores.

Yet, regarding the original biblical recommendation in the Western world this was thought to be hyssop, but in the medieval times and in the time of the Islamic Empire it was known, instead, that the biblical cure isn't hyssop but is, instead, the wild oregano of the Mediterranean mountains. It was only recently re-discovered that this was the case due to the work of the Jewish scholars Fleisher and Fleisher. Investigating herbs growing on the slopes of Mt. Sinai they found no hyssop but, instead, found the wild oregano growing profusely. This proves that wild oregano is the true purging substance mentioned by almighty God. Even so, what does it purge? It primarily purges noxious germs, which overcome the body and ultimately lead to degenerative disease. It also purges the germs which cause sudden infections such as colds, flu, pneumonia, bladder infections, kidney infections, and strep throat.

Yet, for nearly a thousand years humanity neglected it, and as a result suffered inordinate suffering. There were plagues, which were preventable. There were epidemics, which were unnecessary. In fact, there were countless millions of lives which were lost, all of it preventable. This is because if people had truly known about the great lifesaver, the oil of wild oregano, and had merely made use of it and of course made sure of its availability, then the great catastrophes of humanity would have been largely prevented. Even the great 1918 flu epidemic could have been prevented, that is through the vigorous use of spice oils. Regardless, it is little known that this epidemic was largely man-made, as it was a consequence of mass vaccination of military soldiers (see *Cause for Cancer Revealed*). Even so, the oregano would have proven curative and would, therefore, save countless lives. There is much proof of this. For instance, in the United States in one factory the workers were immunized from the flu. So were the workers' family members. These were the cinnamon grinders. The dust from this spice completely protected them from this plague. Yet, too, their family members were protected, because they regularly inhaled the dust from the workers' clothes.

To prove, for instance, the wild oregano's powers there is no need for a so-called double blind study. There is no time for this. The facts are obvious. The scriptures give categorical advice. The only recommendation is for natural substances. Thus, there is seemingly greater wisdom in the ancient scrolls than there is in all of modern medicine. This is because, for instance, the Qur'aan deems pure native honey, like the type which is collected from bees feeding on wild plants, as a medicine, while the Bible holds wild oregano as a powerful cure. Both these medicines have been proven to be more effective than modern antibiotics. Thus, both are obvious recommendations from the loving creator. No human could have recognized these facts, now clearly proven by modern science.

Clearly, as proven historically spice oils are invaluable not only for protecting the human race from dangerous infections but also for reversing existing infections. Too, it is obvious that such information must be popularized, all for the sake of the human race. Those who would inhibit or block this prove by their actions their real motives, which is to put profits and power before the solemn duty to humanity. That duty is, as is memorialized in the Hippocratic Oath, "Above all do no harm." It is a duty which is also codified in the scriptures, for instance, in the Qur'an, where humans are ordained by God only to follow one solemn duty, which is 'to love the fellow human' and in the Bible to 'do unto others as you would have them do unto you.' Both are profound statements that, if practiced, would benefit all humans.

How does this apply to modern times? It surely applies to the operations of the medical profession. Here, financial gain is often placed before human safety. Medicine as a profession is regarded often as a means to wealth. This is especially true in the United States, where there is no restriction on the degree of financial gain a physician can receive. Too, hospitals, mainly private, are motivated by money. The safety and health of the people is usually a secondary consideration. Hospitals are driven by the number of cases they can process, particularly "high end" ones, where insurance pays profusely such as heart disease—especially when the treatment is invasive cardiovascular surgery—and cancer, especially when the treatment involves surgery, chemotherapy, and/or radiation. This is what keeps the hospital "in business." People may be brutally harmed, even killed, to maintain the "profitability" of such centers. Thus, in such instances the warnings of scriptures are disregarded.

Yet, people are living in fear. When a sudden crisis strikes, including a sudden decline health or the development of frightening symptoms, they rush to the doctor. This, while understandable, may lead to such a loss of control that, suddenly, the person may be rushed into surgery or some other invasive treatment. They never have a chance to think about it or to consider other options. Because of the symptoms or the medical findings they are frightened to such a degree that they submit to whatever the physicians command. This is often the case, even before seeking a second opinion.

Or, the person may feel obligated to the physician. He or she may not want to offend the physician and so submits to whatever the doctor declares, even if it makes little or no sense. Yet, here is the rule that all people should follow. People should never submit to others merely to please them. Unless it is an absolute medical emergency, such as, for instance, a proven case of appendicitis, where the appendix is about to burst, or some similar absolute medical crisis—unless the supposed emergency is a true emergency, where there are no other options except massive medical intervention the person should think about it. The person should go home or remove the self from the high-pressure environment. Then, all options should be considered. The possibilities should be investigated. The person should determine if anything natural can be done, that which is safe and non-toxic, that is through diet, exercise, nutritional supplements, and herbal medicine. Can anything non-invasive be done or can the condition be treated without undergoing treatment with dangerous chemicals or radiation? Even with appendicitis the vigorous use of oil of wild oregano sublingually will halt the crisis, without need for surgery. In other words, what safe therapies are available, which never put the person at risk of succumbing to toxicity or side effects?

This is the golden rule. It is also the rule to which all physicians are obliged to submit and to which they agreed under oath during graduation. This is the rule of "Above all do no harm." Yet, it is only the rare physician who abides by this. Furthermore, in the United States and Canada there are no hospitals which hold to this rule, generally being ruled instead by financial motives or, incredibly, mere pride or perhaps arrogance.

Just by doing this, just by taking some time to think about it and to consider other more effective options, countless lives will be saved. The person must consider whether the treatment is sure and if it is indicated. Also, there must be certainty of the correct diagnosis. This is an obvious issue, but the fact is in modern medicine conditions are frequently misdiagnosed. Clearly, if the diagnosis is incorrect, the treatment cannot be appropriate.

This is no attempt for people to defy the doctors. It is merely a simple statement of fact, that is the person should do his or her own homework about the condition before submitting to dangerous treatment, especially when there is no life-threatening emergency. This is because each life is sanctified. This is how God made it, and this is a statement of love for the fellow human and for all humankind.

Regardless, what could be more impressive than the destruction of a drug-resistant germ, and this all achieved by a natural medicine? Here, the wild oregano doesn't discriminate. It kills the regular germs but also the drug resistant type. Moreover, it does so as well as any pharmaceutical agent. Even so, this is no claim to 'replace' drug therapy for this condition with only the oregano. It is merely a statement of fact that is undeniable. This is the fact that the wild oregano achieves a feat that even the most prominent scientists have been unable to achieve. This is the broad spectrum destruction of drug-resistant germs, a function which proves that this invaluable wild spice is one of the most potent and useful substances for the benefit of the human race known.

There is no doubt about it: the wild oregano *is* saving lives. It is now critical to let the world know about it, so that more people can be helped: so that more potential victims can be saved from premature death. Thus, the discovery of the diverse powers of this oil is of even greater importance than the discovery of antibiotics. This is because the wild oregano extract is not only antibacterial but it is also antifungal and antiviral. It is also because this substance reverses the dilemma caused by antibiotics, which is the development and spread of antibiotic resistant germs. Moreover, these are germs which cause countless infections yearly, leading to disfigurement, destruction, and death, most of it preventable. The prevention is in the extensive use of spice oils and spice oil sprays, which must be popularized in modern medicine, all for the sake of the human race.

Chapter Eleven

Conclusion

Spice extracts are the most powerful medicines known. The most powerful of these are the wild spices, particularly wild oregano. Such spices grow wild in the Mediterranean mountains, usually several thousand feet above sea level. The wild oregano was known by the Greeks as *oro ganos*, which means "delight of the mountains." The modern name is merely an Italian corruption of the original Greek. The wild oregano became popular in the United States only since World War II. Soldiers had developed a love for the taste while in the Mediterranean and then, after returning to their country, created the demand for its importation. They could not, it would seem, survive without it.

Today, it would seem impossible for anyone to live without wild oregano. There are so many challenges today, so many stresses. The threats to the human race are high. Many of these threats are microbial. Others are toxic. Still others are venomous. It would be ideal to be prepared for all such threats and be able to ward them off or better yet prevent them. This is through the powers of wild oregano, particularly the high grade steam distilled oil. The ideal therapy is to take the trio of wild oregano products, that is the oil, the crude whole herb plus *Rhus coriaria*, and the essence or juice. For the health of the skin of the hands and face—for the maintenance of this health—the use of the cream is ideal. This may well be the means to extend life in a simple manner. What kills people prematurely? Usually, it is infection. Even with cancer victims rather than the actual tumor it is usually infection, which kills them. In poor countries, often, mere diarrhea kills people. This, too, is due to infection. The elderly frequently die of pneumonia or flu, both of which through the wild oregano therapy are preventable. Let us look at the major killers in, for instance, the United States. Then, the real power of the wild oregano will become clear. These killers are heart disease, stroke, cancer, diabetes, arthritis and its complications, lung disease, the flu, and pneumonia.

Regarding heart disease it is commonly caused by infection as well as inflammation. In this case the infections are low-level, that is chronic. Germs associated with heart disease include nanobacteria, candida, black mold, herpes, strep, staph, and chlamydia. High grade wild oregano oil, Mediterranean source, destroys all these germs. Regarding the inflammation this is due largely because of the infections. By destroying the infections the inflammation is reduced. Even so, as demonstrated by Turkish researchers the wild oregano itself is antiinflammatory. Regarding stroke, this is also often cause by infection, incredibly, by parasites, bacteria, and fungi. Again, the wild oregano either controls or eliminates these infections. Of note, fungi cause a kind of stickiness of the blood, so, in fact, the intake of the oil of wild oregano helps naturally 'thin' or rather normalize the blood. Even so, oil of oregano never causes side effects such as those seen in blood thinners. In fact, if a person is bleeding excessively from a wound the oil of oregano helps halt this. In other words, there is no cause for worry regarding the taking of oil of wild oregano, including with people who have a tendency for strokes. Rather, the intake of the oil, as well as the crude herb and juice, will help prevent this crisis.

People worry needlessly about side effects. The oil of oregano, if from the actual spice, is harmless. In other words, the true food oregano is completely safe for human use, including the oil extract. For instance, in all history there is not a single case of fatality caused by the oil. Nor are there any cases of such a spice oil causing liver or kidney failure. So, why be concerned about it or any supposed side effects? There are fatalities on record from MSG, aspartame, coal tar food dyes, and sulfites. In fact, regarding these substances they have caused thousands of deaths since their introduction. Then, how could anyone even consider oregano as being toxic?

Despite this, people seem to worry endlessly about drug interactions, particularly with any nutritional supplements. Such worry is senseless. For instance, the pharmaceutical industry says oregano is safe. Pharmaceutical agencies list it as a safe substance or food, which has no untoward interactions with medication. Yet, this is true of the true wild oregano, the type that is from the original genetic sources in the deep Mediterranean.

People are afraid of death. They put way too much trust in other humans, notably doctors. Yet, everyone knows that doctors are entirely fallible. So, why place such extreme trust in fallible humans? Would it not be more reliable to trust in the grand Lord of the universe, who is infinite in His powers, while human power is finite? It is such a Being who has made the wild true oregano, which is so helpful and curative, while, in contrast, humans make drugs, which are both destructive and dangerous.

Regardless, rather than considering any noxious effects people should focus on the positive actions. The latter are immense, even endless. After all, the oregano is a key antidote. This is to toxic and allergic reactions. Through this alone countless lives are saved. Plus, it is a full spectrum germicide. This means it is able to kill all known pathogens, including those which cause potentially fatal diseases. Yet, it also kills mutant germs—the drug resistant monsters, which cause great human death and despair. There is no doubt about wild oregano's power, particularly the steam distilled oil, in killing such dangerous mutants.

The oregano oil is the key medicine to rely upon when the unusual or unexpected strikes. Here, it produces dependable results—essentially, it takes the risk out of all that is risky—all that creates fear. Incredibly, this even includes open wounds and venomous bites. It is safe for all these, rather, it is unsafe not to use it. There is no other substance which achieves this diversity of powers.

When antibiotics were first discovered, there was great excitement. The hope for cure was vast. Surely, originally, these antibiotics saved lives. However, soon, their great promise proved disappointing. They did not hold up to the acclaim.

Regarding the value to the human race the high grade wild oregano oil is far more significant than the original antibiotics. More so, it is of greater significance to humanity than all the various antibiotics combined. It is no minor issue that it is mentioned in the ancient scriptures, that is the Old Testament. Thus, it is held high by the almighty God. Yet, there is no national acclaim regarding it? There is no effort by the powerful governments to popularize it. This is despite the fact that such governments have tested it and found it effective. Even so, these same governments under the influence of the major pharmceutical houses accuse those who promote it as hucksters and frauds. No matter what degree of science is presented, still, they deem it valueless.

In 1998 a peculiar event occurred. This was the most unusual attempt by the U.S. government to disprove the power of oil of wild oregano. Under the urging of unknown authorities the FDA set out to prove that oregano was useless. In an unprecedented move the agency hired University of Tennessee Knoxville professor Dr. F. Ann Draughon to demonstrate that the statements about oil of wild oregano were mere quackery. Her method was to test the oregano oil, the original blue- and yellow-label brand, in petri dishes against a wide range of bacteria. She was shocked by the results. The oregano oil obliterated all eight germs against which it was tested, including deadly forms of E. coli and staph. Dr. Draughon disputed the results, claiming laboratory error. After chastising her lab tech she repeated the experiment. There must have been, she made clear, an error: a contaminate—chlorine or some other substance—which was responsible for the results. It couldn't be the oregano. The second experiment proved the same results. Again, all germs were killed. Now, she was really mad and made this clear to her workers. Once again she repeated the results with the same findings. Then, she realized it: it must be the oregano oil.

Dr. Draughon concluded that, while she had presumed that the use of oregano oil or any other spice extract was "useless", without doubt, oregano oil and other spices tested proved to be potent germicides. Her final conclusion was that the oregano should be turned into a drug. Essentially, the U.S. Government accidently proved that oregano oil is more powerful than any other known germ killer. Yet, has anyone heard the slightest mention from the government regarding this?

Even so, the government itself has attempted to profit from wild oregano. This is by patenting a spice oil-based product. This is a food wrap impregnated with oil of oregano and invented by the USDA for purposes of preventing food poisoning. The company which helped spur the government's interest is the maker of the original high-grade oregano oil (blue and yellow label).

As proven by government research, oregano oil, the high mountain variety, destroys a wide range of germs. No antibiotic offers anywhere near this power. As mentioned previously antibiotics only kill categories of germs. For instance, penicillin and ampicillin only kill bacteria, while mycostatin and ketoconazole only kill fungi. Moreover, vaccines kill no germs. Yet, the wild oregano oil kills viruses, bacteria, molds, fungi, and parasites. Moreover, oregano oil has none of the side effects commonly seen in antibiotics such as allergic shock and yeast infections.

Furthermore, some antibiotics only kill a few germs in their category. This is never the case with the wild oil of oregano. When it kills bacteria, it kills nearly every known type, including drug resistant pathogens. Regarding its killing capacity against viruses virtually no virus can resist it. Regarding mold all such germs succumb, as do all yeasts, including the notoriously difficult-to-kill *Candida albicans*. Admittedly, much of this research is in test tubes and animals, yet, regardless, still, in such tests it outperforms any antibiotic. For instance, like oregano oil, mycostatin kills yeasts, but while the former also kills staph, strep, and E. coli the mycostatin has no capacity in this regard. Also, high strength wild oregano oil, as well as multiple spice complexes, destroy toenail and skin fungus and do so more aggressively than any drug.

So, oregano oil is a true miracle. A good grade of this oil made from the wild-growing high mountain spice is a dependable cure, that is for virtually all infectious disease. This is a major issue: to have a reliable cure. It is a substance which can quickly halt an attack of diarrhea, sinusitis, bronchitis, flu, cold, rhinitis, asthma, and gastritis. What else could this be called, other than a cure?

Even so, regarding natural medicine the government doesn't want anyone to use this word. Yet, surgeons claim to cure. For instance, cardiovascular surgeons, after performing open heart surgery, claim to cure their patients. These surgeons may freely claim the power to cure, even though they lack any true scientific studies about their procedures. For instance, with heart by-pass surgery there is no evidence that such a procedure is curative, rather, in many instances it proves fatal. In contrast, consider the use of oil of oregano in, for instance, angina. Here, it often eliminates the angina, and it does so more rapidly and effectively than any drug. Consider, too, its powers in colds and flu, where it can obliterate all symptoms—where it categorically destroys all traces of the cold/flu viruses—in mere minutes. Regarding bronchial and sinus conditions, here, also, it is supreme. In such conditions, where no drug can help, the oregano oil gives not only relief but ultimately reverses these conditions. With diarrhea it may halt all symptoms in mere minutes. Then, with such a phenomenal substance the entire medical world should categorically reveal it. Yet, instead, all is done that is possible to resist it.

Yet, in contrast to drugs it is the oregano oil which is lifesaving. This oil alone destroys entire categories of life-threatening infections. E. coli, staph, strep, clostridium, klebsiella, proteus, and hemophilus all succumb to it. It is also this oil which people depend upon to avoid common illnesses. It is this oil which countless thousands of people depend upon when traveling to prevent any crisis. Yet, how was this discovered? It was discovered by the people on their own, without any guidance from the medical community. People determined its powers by using it and gaining the countless benefits. No one helped them understand it. They found out on their own through their own experience.

Since wild oregano is a lifesaving spice, the information about it must not be suppressed. Those who do so are guilty of a great crime. This is the crime of neglect, where people in need could be helped—but that help is maliciously denied to them.

There is much reason to hold wild oregano and other natural medicines high. The great scriptures mention natural cures as a gift to the human race. The Qur'aan dedicates an entire section to the bee, describing its production, honey, as a "medicine for humankind." This book also indicates that pomegranate and olive oil have medicinal properties. The Bible also mentions honey; it is well known that the great men of this scripture, Jacob, Joseph, Solomon, and David, were fond of it. Jesus surely recommended it, as "strong ointment", that its strength was surely being derived from heat-producing plants such as wild oregano. The latter was the main medicinal plant growing in the mountains during the time of Jesus.

Yet, of all scriptures it is the Bible which has the actual specific recommendation. It is this text alone which urges human beings to use specifically wild oregano. Also, as mentioned previously the Prophet Muhammad strongly recommended it, telling his followers to take it internally and also use it in the home, possibly burning it as incense. Then, the basis of this is now known, since this powerful spice reverses an enormous number of ailments, particularly those caused by infections. It is as if the great God wishes His human race to be well to such a degree that He specifically tells them what to take, even specifying the exact spice, which is most powerful—just as He recommends specifically in the Qur'aan raw honey as a health-aid.

There are a number of wild oregano products that a person can utilize. There is the crude wild oregano herb, with its companion wild herb, *Rhus coriaria*. This is an ideal supplement for daily use and is a key formula for the health of the digestive tract. There is the oil of wild oregano, which is extracted from the wild oregano leaves through steam distillation. This is the basic germicide and is the primary wild oregano supplement. It is ideally taken as drops under the tongue, although gelatin capsules are also available. Regarding sudden or chronic infections this is the best type to use.

Too, there is the essence, which is also a steam extract. This essence or juice is the oxygenated drink, which is ideal for the nervous system. It is usually found in health food stores in a brown amber 12-ounce bottle. A typical dose is a tablespoon or two daily. There is also the cold extract, made through infusing carbon dioxide under pressure through the raw herb, this being an ideal natural medicine for chronic viral infections and also ideal for use topically against warts. This is also the type to use for 'suspicious' skin lesions. It is available usually as a one-ounce dropper bottle

A wild oregano oil-based cream with propolis, Canada balsam, honey, wild lavender oil, and wild St. John's wort is the ideal wild oregano product for skin conditions. Such a cream is particularly potent for the health of the skin of the face and hands. It can be used as a 'sun-block' but, more importantly, for reversing sun-induced damage. There is great power in this cream, as it is a totally natural emollient for skin health. The cream is, thus, a must for the prevention of skin aging. In this respect, ideally, it should be applied daily. It is so natural that it is edible. Thus, it is free of all synthetic chemicals.

For children there is a special type, which is water soluble. It blends perfectly in milk or any fatty drink but also blends well in juice. It is not as hot as the regular oil of oregano and, thus, is more well tolerated by children. This type may also be used in the treatment of pets and can be added to food and water. It is safe for all ages and is known as mycelized oil of oregano. There is also a water soluble wild oregano spray. This spray contains other natural spice oils such as oils of clove, bay leaf, and cumin. Such sprays are effective in reducing or eliminating germ counts in air. They can also be used on hard surfaces to reduce germ counts. In addition, wild oregano-based sprays may be used as throat sprays or may be sprayed in sick rooms or added to vaporizers. Incredibly, such sprays also act as natural bug repellents.

So, wild oregano and other spice oil-based products are the most important natural medicines for the home medicine chest. While drugs cause innumerable side effects the oregano is free of any such toxicity. In contrast to drugs it never causes fatality, rather, it prevents deaths. This is an impressive statement—that rather than highly touted drugs it is a natural substance which is the real weapon against disease. While vaccines and drugs cause obvious deaths wild oregano oil clearly saves lives. Surely, there are thousands of people alive today who would otherwise surely be dead, or be crippled, if it weren't for the wild oregano. Perhaps this is why it is such a threat.

Even so, there is no amount of proof that could be provided which would cause any opponents to accept this. The information in this book will always be resisted, especially by the established medical authorities. This is a threat to the medical system, because this one natural medicine makes obsolete hundreds of medical therapies and procedures. Even if scientific studies are performed proving beyond any doubt the diverse powers of oil of wild oregano, still, it will be resisted.

Consider peoples' testimonies. Typically, this is "disallowed" by the government powers. In this regard there is great policing by the government against the use of such testimony. Yet, essentially, a person's testimony is like a medical case. This is known in medicine as a clinical case. It is a kind of initial proof or evidence of the potential power of a treatment. In medicine and surgery this is acceptable as evidence. Thus, for natural or nutritional treatments this, too, must be regarded as valid, as long as it is true and sincere. It may not be final proof, yet, it is a good part of it and, thus, must never be disregarded.

What more proof is needed? If a person is suffering from a health crisis and, then, takes the oil of wild oregano—and the crisis is halted—this is proof. There is no basis to reject this. Regardless, the basis of accepted 'cures' is no better: supposed double blind studies. Yet, these 'studies' are done by the drug companies themselves, and the majority of these have recently been shown to be fabricated. Moreover, the fabrication is intentional. The proof of this is found in Marcia Angell's

The Truth about the Drug Companies. Angell states categorically that it is the goal of these companies to deceive the public in every way possible in order to achieve market goals.

Then, since the research is bogus real stories of human benefits are far more revealing. That is correct: an accurate testimonial from an afflicted person who, then, finds benefit in a natural substance and who documents this—in fact, this is more useful than fabricated studies. Thus, people can surely focus on the testimonials. They are a means to truly learn the powers of the wild oregano. They are a tool to give confidence for treating and reversing virtually any condition. They are also a tool to motivate, so a person will confidently take the appropriate therapy for his or her needs. It is inspiring to have this information, these real life cases of how people in despair are helped by a God-given spice. Not only were are they helped, but also many of the people have found their lives lengthened and their paths made easy: all through the powers of natural cures.

People aren't stupid. Nor do they seek to lie regarding such critical information. The general population takes the giving of endorsements seriously. Thus, people report their testimonies, essentially, in a conservative manner. Thus, again, make use of the testimonies as a guide for the use of wild oregano and other spice extracts.

The history of wild oregano is proof both of its use and power. No one can deny it: the human race has consistently relied upon this potent spice for the better health and also for the cure of disease. The fact that this is mentioned in the earliest of divine books is surely impressive. The Sumerian and Babylonian use is also a significant issue, as these societies recorded its value in a wide range of illnesses, including lung and bronchial complaints, infected wounds, battle wounds, and heart disease. As mentioned previously the Prophet of Islaam regarded it highly, deeming it a cure for the common cold. This has been borne true by modern research as well as actual human results. The Bible's claim has also been demonstrated as true, which is that the wild oregano purges the body of poisons and toxins—and these poisons/toxins include all manner of noxious germs. More recently, British herbalists, 1500s through the 1600s, held wild oregano highly. They deemed the oil as a cure for diarrheal and stomach diseases such as those caused by food and water poisoning. Also, oregano oil was held as the most powerful treatment for colds and earaches. For tuberculosis they claimed the watery essence (steam extract) as curative.

There are a number of natural medicines that are ideal for health regeneration. These are the oil of wild oregano, the whole crude herb with *Rhus coriaria*, the oregano-treated wild raw triple greens flushing agent, and the wild raw eight berries cleansing/rebuilding complex.

For many people, especially those who have a heavy load of toxins in their bodies, those who have been continuously exposed to poisonous substances in food, water, and air, a purge may be necessary. This is through the intake of a natural edible oil, wild greens, and spice oil purging formula. This formula is ideal for cleansing poisons from the liver, gallbladder, and blood. The cleansing occurs through the stool and urine. There is no 'laxative' action of such a formula. Rather, this is a systematic cleansing for the removal of poisonous substances. It can be easily taken under a full schedule. There is no need to stay away from work. For best results take this purge along with the aforementioned therapeutic program. The purge helps reestablish normal liver function, which is essential for all bodily functions. It is to be taken as a daily dose in the morning, about an ounce, for at least 24 days. Each bottle would ideally contain 12 ounces. The most potent ingredients of such a purge would include extra virgin olive oil, remote-source black seed oil, organic apple cider vinegar, wild raw nettles extract, wild raw burdock leaf extract, wild raw dandelion leaf extract, wild raw clintonia leaf extract, wild raw fireweed extract, wild raw high bush cranberry extract, along with various spice oils.

Also, the immune system must be boosted with the necessary vitamins. The key vitamins for the immune system are the B complex, vitamin C, and vitamin A. The B complex is found in coarse whole grains, brown rice, wild rice, organic liver, wholesome/grass-fed red meat, poultry, organic cheese, whole organic milk, and dark green leafy vegetables.

Regarding concentrates that are easy to take there is rice polish, wild raw greens drops, the latter being rich in the difficult-to-procure riboflavin, and brewer's yeast. There are, thus, very few foods which are top sources of this group of vitamins. For vitamin A the best sources are cod liver oil, organic liver, and red sockeye salmon oil. Of these, the red sockeye salmon oil is the purest. Thus, for the immune system as a source of natural vitamin A this may be consumed on a daily basis, either as a whole oil by the teaspoon or fish gelatin capsules. The vitamin A is a key substance for strengthening the entire immune system. Thus, natural-source vitamin A must be included in any wild oregano therapy program.

Vitamin C is also critical. The key with this vitamin is to consume it on a regular basis, since it is water soluble and it is readily lost from the body. Moreover, it should be consumed both in foods and whole food concentrates. Ideal food sources include lemons, limes, grapefruit, oranges, strawberries, broccoli, dandelion greens, and papaya. To reverse disease natural vitamin C is far more potent than the synthetic type. This is the ideal type to use with the oregano therapy. The combination of natural vitamin C concentrates plus wild oregano is a potent therapy. The most dense source of natural vitamin C is concentrates of camu camu, rose hips, and acerola. This concentrate is as a bulk powder or as capsules. The vitamin C helps boost white blood cell activity. It also strengthens the cellular tissues. This is by aiding in the formation in a kind of cellular cement. Cells that are well connected through this cement are highly immunized against attack by germs.

Truly natural vitamin C serves several critical functions. It helps boost the function of the immune cells, helping keep them in the most active state possible. White cells lacking this vitamin become sluggish. It also is needed to increase the production of key immune proteins known as immunoglobulins. Furthermore, as mentioned previously the vitamin is needed to strengthen the internal tissues, particularly the tissues known as the connective tissues. With strong connective tissues there is a high resistance against the invasion of germs as well as cancer.

Ideally, the natural source vitamin C complex should be taken at the same time as taking the wild oregano. For best results this vitamin C complex, which consists of a combination of wild camu camu, acerola cherry, and rose hips, should be taken at least twice daily. This will help maintain blood levels of this delicate compound, which is readily lost from the body. Vitamin C stays in the body a relatively short time. So, for optimal health it must be continuously replenished. Even so, the natural source type is retained by the body far more readily than the synthetic type, which is quickly lost into the urine. At a minimum the aforementioned natural substances, along with the purge, must be taken for the creation of ideal health. The combination of the wild raw greens and berries, along with the oregano, is far superior to taking the oregano alone. The metabolic type is also critical. For more information about how each person can find their type see the novel book *Eat Right for Your Hormone System* (same author, Knowledge House Publishers). Here, a person will learn the status of his/her endocrine system, which is a highly crucial finding. The endocrine system exerts massive control over health. By discovering the type and, then, balancing the system there will be an overall improvement in health. For those who suffer from chronic disease as well as all who suffer from chronic infections there are great benefits from balancing this system.

The body type is based upon an inherent metabolic weakness. The main four types are the thyroid, adrenal, pituitary, and combination, that is thyroid-adrenal or pituitary-adrenal, types. To have a type means that the involved organ(s) is/are weak and therefore must be strengthened for health improvement. For instance, thyroid and pituitary types are vulnerable to fungal infections, while adrenal types are vulnerable to viral infections as well as tuberculosis.

Thus, there is no attempt to proclaim oregano or other spices as cure-alls. To achieve optimal health a number of approaches must be pursued. Healthy diet, proper exercise, fresh air, relaxation, and natural cleansing are all part of a get healthy plan. Even so, the wild oregano in particular offers great power with rapid results in countless conditions. This is particularly true in acute infections, yet it is also largely true in chronic infections. It is also true in many instances of pain and inflammation. What's more, the wild oregano is a reliable cure in a wide range of sudden crises, such as an attack by a venomous creature, potentially infected wounds, allergic shock, blood poisoning, and infectious diarrhea. There are virtually no medical treatments for such potentially disastrous, as well as fatal, crises.

Again, for healing the body, especially in the event of chronic debilitating disease, a systematic approach must be taken. In essence there must be both cleansing and killing. Thus, the combination of the wild oregano plus the wild raw greens and berries is most effective. This is because while the wild oregano kills any invasive or dangerous germs the wild raw greens and berries extracts cleanse the tissues of toxins. The combination is ideal for the creation of great energy and power. To reiterate, three key supplements are the wild oregano, both as the whole herb and the oil, the wild triple greens extract, with wild burdock, nettles, and dandelion, and the wild maximum strength raw berry extract taken as drops under the tongue. Virtually anyone can gain an improvement in health through the intake of these most potent substances.

Yet, this is only the case with the pure whole food form of oregano, the type which grows wild in the high Mediterranean mountains. This is the type thoroughly investigated by prominent scientific studies such as those listed in this book. It is also the type which has been used by humankind for countless years, the type specifically recommended in divine script. Furthermore, this makes sense, since the wild growing material is far more potent than any farm-raised or human corrupted type.

Even so, there are numerous attempts to corrupt wild oregano and even to, incredibly, patent it. For instance, through funding received from the U. S. government the University of Massachusetts has actually patented a form of fabricated 'oregano.' This university actually initially contacted me to gain my help. Said the proponents, "Would you help us market our product?", that is their specific *genetically engineered* oregano. The initial interest to use oregano was, of course, stimulated through the original book on the subject, *The Cure is in The Cupboard*. In this book only wild naturally occurring oregano is recommended. The university received money derived from taxpayers to produce their own patented form of oregano. So, since the government is invested in oregano, obviously, any attempt to impugn it is bogus.

The fact is nature is the greatest of all healers. This is the source of many of the most commonly used pharmaceutical drugs. It is the source of numerous anti-cancer drugs. It is the source of aspirin and digoxin, the latter being used for the prevention of heart disorders. It is the source of numerous antibiotics, including penicillin, mycostatin, and amphotericin. It is also the source of the most powerful germ killer known, wild oregano.

Too, there is the issue of the revelations regarding oregano by the USDA. It was S. Wang, a biochemist at the government's Beltsville Agricultural Center, who stated that the oregano herb was "3 to 20 times higher" in antioxidant activity than the other herbs tested. This meant that the whole oregano herb was some 4 to 5 times more powerful as an antioxidant than blueberries.

Thus, wild oregano, particularly the steam-extracted oil, is highly versatile. It is a potent antiseptic plus it is one of the most powerful antioxidants known. It contains significant pain killing and, therefore, antiinflammatory activity. The oil of wild oregano is the ideal natural antifungal agent, as it kills all types of fungi, including yeasts and molds. It is also the ideal antibiotic-like substance, because it kills the complete range of bacteria. As an antiviral agent it is unmatched, as no virus can resist its powers. As an antiparasitic it is also invaluable, since it kills a significant range of such invaders, particularly amebas and protozoans. The whole crude herb is a top source of natural flavonoids as well as minerals and vitamins. This is significant proof that whole foods, including whole unprocessed spices, are the medicines of the future.

So, let it be known. As revealed by almighty God wild oregano has vast curative powers. This master of the universe has given humanity this blessed spice as a gift. This is a lifesaving spice. It is the most potent natural medicine known. Moreover, because of its exclusively positive effects on the human body it is invaluable for the human race.

Bibliography

Adam, K., et al. 1998. Antifungal activities of *Origanum vulgare* subsp. *hirtum, Mentha spicata, Lavandula angustifolia,* and *Salvia fruticosa* essential oils against human pathogenic fungi. *J. Agric. Food Chem.* 46: 1739-1745.

Alma, H. M., et al. 2003. Screening chemical composition and in vitro antioxidant and antimicrobial activities of the essential oils from *Origanum syriacum* L. growing in Turkey. *Biological & Pharmaceutical Bulletin.* 26:1725-29.

Asil, E., Tanker, M., and S. Sar. 1984. Headache folk remedies used in central Anatolia region. *J. Fac. Pharm. Ankara.* 14:67-80.

Atanda, O. O., Akpan, I., and F. Oluwafemi. 2006. The potential of some essential oils in the control of *Aflatoxin parasiticus* CFR 223 and aflatoxin production. *Food Cont.* 18:601.

Aydin, S., et al. 1996. Investigation of Origanum onites, Sideritis congesta, and Satureja cuneifolia essential oils for analgesic activity. *Phytotherapy Research.*

Aydin, S., Ozturk, Y., and K.H.C. Baser. 1997. Cardiovascular actions of Kekik (Origanum onites L.) essential oil. *Proc. XIth Symp. Origin. Crude Drugs* (Ankara). May, pp. 339-344.

Aydin, S. and E. Seker. 2005. Effect of an aqueous distillate of Origanum onites L. on isolated rat fundus, duodenum, and ileum: evidence for the role of oxygenated monoterpenes. *Pharmazie.* 60:147-150.

Becerril, R., et al. 2007. Combination of analytical and microbiological techniques to study the antimicrobial activity of a new active food packaging containing cinnamon or oregano against E. coli and S. aureus. *Anal Bioanal. Chem.* 388:1003.

Bendini, A., Toschi Gallina, T., and C. Lercker. 2002. Antioxidant activity of oregano (*Origanum vulgare*) leaves. *Ital. J. Food. Sci.* 14:17-24.

Bennis, S., et al. 2004. Surface alteration of Saccharomyces cerevisiae induced by thymol and eugenol. *Letters Appl. Micro.* 38:454.

Braga, P. C., et al. 2006. Anti-inflammatory activity of thymol: inhibitory effect on the release of human neutrophil elastase. *Pharmacology*. 77:130-136.

Burkowski, Al, et al. 2007. Effects of a combination of thyme and oregano essential oils on TNBS-induced colitis in mice. *Hindawi Publishing Corp.* Article ID: 23296.

Burt, S. A. and R. D. Reiners. 2003. Antibacterial activity of selected plant essential oils against Escherichia coli 0157:H7. *Letters in Applied Microbiology*. 36:162.

Burt, S. 2004. Essential oils: their antibacterial properties and potential applications in foods a review. *Int. J. Food Microbiol*. 94:223-253.

Caillet, S., Shareck, F. and M. Lacroix. 2005. Effect of gamma radiation and oregano essential oil on murein and ATP concentration of Escherichia coli. 157:H7. *J. Food Prot*. 68:2571-79.

Chamil, N., et al. 2004. Antifungal treatment with carvacrol and eugenol of oral candidiasis in immuunosuppressed rats. *Brazilian Journal of Infectious Diseases*. 8:217-226.

Culpepper's Complete Herbal. Exeter: W. Foulsham & Co.

Donaldson, J. R., et al. 2005. Assessment of antimicrobial activity of fourteen essential oils when using dilution and diffusion methods. *Pharmaceutical Biology*. 43: 687.

Dorman, H. J. D. and S. G. Davies. 2000. Antimicrobial agents from plants: antibacterial activity of plant volatile oils. *J. Appl. Micro*. 88:306.

Elgayyar, M., Draughon, F. A., Golden, D. A., and J. R. Mount. 2001. Antimicrobial activity of plant volatile oils. *J. Food Prot*. 64:1019-1024.

Essawi, T. and M. Srour. 2000. Screening of some Palestinian medicinal plants for antibacterial activity. *J. Ethnopharm*. 70:343.

Florou-Paneri, P., et al. 2005. Oregano herb verus oregano essential oil as feed supplements to increase the oxidative stability of turkey meat. *International Journal of Poultry Science*. 4:866.

Force, M. Sparks, W. S. and R. A. Ronzio. 2000. Inhibition of enteric parasites by emulsified oil of oregano in vivo. *Phytotherapy Research*. 14:213-0214.

Grieve, M. 1992. *A Modern Herbal*. Great Britain: Cresset Press.

Hammer, K. A., Carson, C. F., and T. V. Riley. 1999. Antimicrobial activity of essential oils and other plant extracts. *J. Appl. Micro.* 86:985.

Helms, M., Vastrup, P., Gerner-Smidt, P., and K. Molbak. 2003. Short and long term mortality associated with foodborne bacterial gastrointestinal infections: registry based study. *British Medical Journal.* 326:357.

Hideyuki, M., et al. 2003. DPPH radical scavengers from dried leaves of oregano (*Origanum vulgare*). *Biosci. Biotechnol. Biochem.* 67:2311.

Ijaz, K. M., et al. 2004. Antiviral and virucidal activities of Oregano P73-based spice extracts against human coronavirus in vitro. *Antiviral Research* (abstract), presented at: Seventeenth International Conference on Antiviral Research.

Ingram, C. 2008. *The Cure is in the Cupboard: How to Use Oregano for Better Health.* Buffalo Grove, IL: Knowledge House Publishers.

Ingram, C. 2003. *The Respiratory Solution.* Buffalo Grove, IL: Knowledge House Publishers.

Ipek, E., Zeytinoglu, H., Okay, S., Tuylu, B. A., Kurkcuoglu, M., and K. Husnu Can Baser. 2004. Genotoxicity and antigenotoxicity of Origanum oil and carvacrol evaluated by Ames Salmonella/microsomal test. *Analytical, Nutritional and Chemical Methods* (Feb).

Juglala, S., et al. 2002. Spice oils for the control of co-occurring mycotoxin-producing fungi. *J. Food Prot.* 65:683.

Kalemba, D. and A. Kunicka. 2003. Antibacterial and antifungal properties of essential oils. *Current Microbiology Chemistry.* 10: 813.

Lambert, R. J. W., Skandamis, P. N., Coote, P. J., and G. J. E. Nychas. 2001. A study of the minimum inhibitory concentration and mode of action of oregano essential oil, thymol, and carvacrol. *Journal of Applied Microbiology.* 91:453.

Lima, I. O., et al. 2005. Inhibitory action of some phytochemicals on yeasts potentially causing opportunistic infections. *Rev. Bras. Clen. Farm.* 41:199.

Lin, Y. T., Lahbe, R. G., and Kalidas Shetty. 2004. Inhibition of Listeria monocytogenes in fish and meat systems by use of oregano and cranberry phytochemical synergies. *Applied and Environmental Microbiology.* 70:5672.

Manohar, V., Ingram, C., Gray, J., et al. 2001. Antifungal activities of origanum oil against Candida albicans. *Molecular and Cellular Biochemistry.* 228:111-117.

Martinez-Tome, M., Jimenez, A. M., Ruggieri, S., Frega, N., Strabbioli, R., and M. A. Murcia. 2001. Antioxidant properties of Mediterranean spices compared with common food additives. *J. Food Prot.* 64:1412-1419.

Misha, N., Upman, K., and D. Shulka. 2000. Antifungal activity of essential oil of *Cinnamonium zeylanicum*. *J. Essential Oil Research.* 3:97-110.

Mohacsi-Farkas, C., Tulok, M., and B. Balogh. Antimicrobial Activity of Greek Oregano and Winter Savory Extracts (Essential Oil and SCFE) Investigated by Impedimetry. *Acta Horticulturae* 597, International Conference on Medicinal and Aromatic Plants (Part III).

Nostro, A., et al. 2004. Susceptibility of methicillin-resistant staphylococci to oregano essential oil, carvacrol, and thymol. *FEMS Microbiol. Lett.* 230:191-195.

Ozcan, M. 2005. Effect of spice hydrosols on the growth of Aspergillus parasiticus NRRL 2999 strain. *J. Med. Food.* 8:275.

Pattnaik, S., Subramanyan, V.R., and C. Kole. 1996. Antibacterial antifungal activity of ten essential oils in vitro. *Microbios.* 86:121-126.

Preuss, H. G., et al. 2005. Effects of essential oils and monolaurin on *Staphylococcus aureus*: In vitro and in vivo studies. *Toxicology Mechanism and Method.* 15:279.

Ramzi, A. A., et al. 2008. Antimicrobial, antioxidant, and cytotoxic activities and phytochemical screening of some Yemeni medicinal plants. *Evidence-Based Complementary and Alternative Medicine.*

Sivropoulou, A., et al. 1996. Antimicrobial and cytotoxic activities of Origanum essential oils. *J. Agric. Food Chem.* 44:1200-1205.

Skandamis, P., et al. 2001. Inhibition of oregano essential oil and EDTA on Escherichia coli 0157:H7. *Ital. J. Food Sci.* 13:65.

Sokovic, M., et al. 2002. Antifungal activities of selected aromatic plants growing wild in Greece. *Nahrung.* (Oct):317-320.

Soliman, K. M. and R. I. Badeae. 2002. Effect of oil extracted from some medicinal plants on different mycotoxigenic fungi. *Food Chem. Toxicol.* 144:1669.

Soylu, S., Yigitbas, H., Soylu, E.M., and S. Kurt. 2007. Antifungal effect of essential oils from oregano and fennel on Sclerotinia sclerotiorum. *J. Appl. Micro.* 103:1021-1030.

Srihari, T., Sengottuvelan, M., and N. Nalina. 2008. Dose-dependent effect of oregano (Origanum vulgare L.) on lipid peroxidation and antioxidant status in 1,2-dimethyhydrazine-induced rat colon carcinogenisis. *Pharm. Pharmacol.* 60:787-794.

Ultee, A., Kets, E. P. W., and E. J. Smid. 1999. Mechanism of action of carvacrol on the food-borne pathogen Bacillus cereus. *Appl. Enviro. Micro.* 65:4606-4610.

Ulukanli, Z., et al. 2005. Antimicrobial activities of some plants from the eastern Anatolia region of Turkey. *Pharmaceutical Biology.* 43:334-339.

Uyanoglu, M., et al. Effect of carvacrol upon the liver of rats undergoing partial hepatectomy. *Phytomedicine.* 15:226.

Wilcox, J. K., Ash, S. L., and G. L. Catignani. 2004. Antioxidants and prevention of chronic disease. *Crit. Rev. Food Sci. Nutr.* 44:275-295.

Index

A

Alzheimer's disease, 16, 32, 164
Acne, 15, 32, 170
Addison's disease, 50
AIDS, 22
Air
    purification of, 93–98
Allergic reactions, 7, 28–29, 224
Allergic rhinitis, 50, 129, 154
ALS. *See* Lou Gehrig's Disease
Angell, Marcia, 194–195, 231–232
Ankylosing spondylitis, 50
Ant repellent, 81
Antibiotics, 7–8, 21, 23, 45–48, 69,
    77, 98, 100, 103, 105, 128, 155,
    207–208, 216, 220, 224, 226, 238
Antifungal diet, 44, 134–135
Anxiety neurosis, 50
Arthritis, 21, 31, 49, 75, 108, 123,
    126, 129, 167, 173, 182, 187, 200,
    213, 222
Asthma, 31, 36–37, 50, 58, 68, 85–86,
    95, 123, 129, 137, 141, 149, 154–155,
    173, 227
Attention deficit disorder, 50, 108,
Autism, 34, 50, 108, 124, 129
Autoimmune thyroiditis, 50

B

Back pain, 81
Bacteria, 10–16, 27–28, 46, 51, 90, 94,
    98–99, 103, 125, 129, 145, 148–152,
    155, 170, 174–176, 207–209, 212,
    222, 225–226, 239
Bay leaf oil, 11–12, 23, 42–44, 49, 52,
    53, 60, 73, 79–80, 96–98, 128, 134,
    136, 138, 154, 163, 172, 230
Bee sting, 28–29, 85
    see also Wasp sting
Bile, 26–27, 114, 131, 187
Black seed oil, 26–27, 31, 78, 131,
    133, 138, 234
Blood clots, 84–85
Bowel cleansing, 25
Bronchitis, 50, 58, 63, 95, 106, 129, 137,
    154, 155, 227
Burns, 168–169, 197, 203

C

Cancer, 31, 34, 36, 49, 72, 83, 88, 93,
    108, 123, 151–162, 174, 188, 190,
    213–217, 222, 235, 238
Candida, 36, 39, 58, 97, 122, 143–144,
    222, 226
    see also Yeast infection; Fungal infection
Carvacrol, 21, 115–116, 120, 144, 153,
    160, 162, 180–181
Case histories
    allergy, 85
    ALS, 124
    ant repellent, 81
    asthma, 68, 85-86
    autism, 131–132
    bee sting, 85
    blood clots, 84–85
    bronchitis, 106–107

Additional Health Books from
Knowledge House Publishers

How to Eat Right and Live Longer
Softcover 361 pages–$24.95 #022

You can lose weight, increase your energy, normalize your blood pressure, wipe out headaches, and even eliminate disease, all by eating right. Find out what the real time bombs are and eliminate them from the diet. Determine how you can live longer, just by changing shopping habits. Take the diet tests to find out what is poisoning you and how to correct it. Includes a special section, For Doctors Only, plus protocols and over 100 recipes.

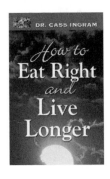

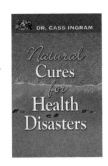

Nutrition Tests for Better Health
Softcover 355 pages–$24.95 #035

Discover your body's nutritional needs before you supplement. Know what you should eat and what supplements you need based upon your personal test scores. Determine the specific nutritional and hormonal needs of your body—your vitamin and mineral deficiencies, plus any imbalances in hormones, metabolism, and the immune system. Plus, this book provides information on the dosages and types of vitamins and minerals needed for optimal health.

Natural Cures for Health Disasters
Soft cover 384 pages–$24.95 #2000

Cure any health disaster from A to Z. Learn which foods, herbs, spices, and oils reverse dozens of illnesses and injuries, including skin disorders, allergic attacks, infections, asthma, wounds, swelling, pain, exposure to toxins, and dozens more. This is your home bible for staying safe and also getting the help you need, regardless of the crisis. Includes specific protocols for dozens of ailments and diseases.

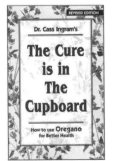

The Cure is in the Cupboard
Softcover 210 pages–$19.95 #016

Newly revised, this best-seller is the book of protocols for exactly how to use wild oreganoto treat over 100 ailments. Read about what ancient scriptures call the "purging" spice.This is the how-to guide for dozens of disorders, including sinus problems, respiratory conditions, bacterial and fungal infections, winter illnesses, and more.

Natural Cures for Killer Germs
Softcover 384 pages–$19.95 #2003

Killer germs are everywhere. Learn how to protect
yourself so you are not a victim. Also, learn the role of
vaccinations in introducing killer germs into the body.
The history of the polio vaccine and its dangers are
revealed. Learn about the cover-up. Are you a victim?
Read the connection of contaminated vaccines to MS,
ALS, Parkinson's disease, and immune deficiency.
Protocols on dozens of diseases, including H. Pylori,
MRSA, TB, hepatitis C, and flu, are included.

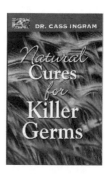

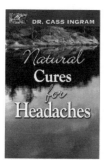

Natural Cures for Headaches
Softcover 230 pages–$18.95 #9027

Dr. Ingram proves the headache connection of toxic
foods, food additives, and chemicals. Discover the role
of heavy metals, hormonal imbalances, dental fillings,
nutritional deficiencies, chronic infections, and drug
toxicity, and how to naturally correct them. The cause of
headaches can be found and reversed without drugs. A
special herbal formula which rapidly eliminates
migraines is included.

Natural Cures for Diabetes
Softcover 330 pages–$19.95 #9029

You can reverse your diabetes naturally by treating the
cause. Learn about the enormous role of nutritional
deficiency in this disease. Find out which foods, spices,
and herbs act as natural insulin. Get specific protocols
for all types of diabetes plus complications and
additional information for reversing low blood sugar.
Includes recipes, and three week eating right menu.

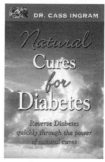

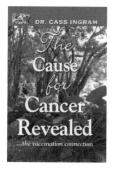

The Cause for Cancer Revealed
Softcover 350 pages–$22.95 #9030

Dr. Ingram reveals the connection between animal
viruses, vaccinations, and cancer. He also tells how
natural medicines can reverse, even cure, today's most
deadly disease. He describes the vaccine danger, as
well as the cure. Determine your risks for developing
cancer and discover the natural medicines you can use
to treat and even cure it.

The Longevity Solution
Softcover 136 pages–$13.95 #2001

Here is proof about the only documented substance in nature known to extend life. Learn how you can dramatically improve your energy and strength with natural royal jelly supplements. Also read about real medicinal honey and the power of bee propolis. Find out how to use royal jelly concentrate to improve your appearance and, most of all, to live a healthy and long life.

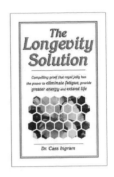

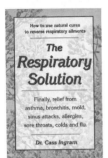

The Respiratory Solution
Softcover 157 pages–$14.95 #2002

This is the solution to your respiratory problems, whether sinus, bronchial, or lung. Find out the real cause of chronic respiratory conditions, including asthma, bronchitis, and sinusitis. Learn the role of fungi and yeasts in lung conditions. Find out the importance of sleeping on the right side and the power of breathing exercises. Includes exact protocols of diet and supplements for the reversal of these conditions.

SuperMarket Remedies
Hardcover 330 pages–$29.95 #031

Food is medicine. You can prevent illness and cure yourself with what you eat. Begin your search for preventing or curing illness in the supermarket/health food store. Dr. Ingram informs you about foods which fight everyday ailments, stop pain, and save you money; for instance, a spice that eliminates cold/flu symptoms faster than drugs, and a luscious fruit that lowers cholesterol rapidly.

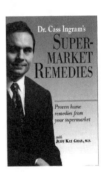

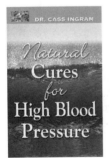

Natural Cures for High Blood Pressure
Softcover 330 pages–$19.95 #9028

Reverse high blood pressure, plus numerous other heart/arterial diseases, without drugs. Learn about the nutritional connection to high blood pressure. Also, discover the dental connection to this illness. Determine the infection connection to high blood pressure and how to reverse it. Learn how exotic oils, such as sesame and black seed, can reverse this disease. Also includes recipes.

Tea Tree Oil: The Natural Antiseptic
Softcover 119 pages–$13.95 #080

Learn all the uses for tea tree oil to keep the body healthy. This is the topical antiseptic and antitoxin that can be lifesaving. It is antifungal, antibacterial, and antiviral; learn how to use it for injuries, skin conditions, scalp disorders, acne boils, toothaches, athlete's foot, and much more. Works well with oil of wild oregano.

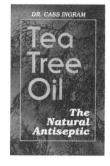

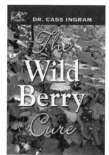

The Wild Berry Cure
Softcover 248 pages–$19.95 #9012

Learn the secret powers of wild raw berry extracts. Also learn the power of wild raw berries and how they can increase energy, muscular strength, cleanse toxins, reduce excess weight, rebuild all the body functions plus, improve the tone and beauty of skin as well as hair. Also helps with heart disease, diabetes, arthritis, brain and nerve conditions, cancer, and much more.

The Warning Signs of Nutritional Deficiency—Kit
Contains: handboook and your choice of 4 CDs or casettes–$89.95 #097

Know the Warning signs to determine exactly what the body needs. This is the ideal tool for improving diagnostic ability. For nutritional deficiency the face, skin, nails, and hair are revealing. Certain signs also reveal hormonal status. Routine blood work reveals specific nutritional deficiencies and glandular imbalances—all based upon published literature. Nutritional zrecommendations as well as tests and case histories (for personal study) are included. Find out what your body needs nutritionally. Ideal for health professionals.

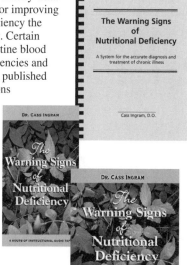

KNOWLEDGE HOUSE PUBLISHERS   ORDER FORM

BOOK #	TITLE	QTY	$ AMOUNT

Make checks payable to:
Knowledge House Publishers
105 East Townline Road.
Unit 116,
Vernon Hills, IL 60061

www.knowledgehousepublishers.com
1-866-626-5888
fax-1-847-473-4780
for email inquiries:
info@knowledgehousepublishers.com

For American Express, Visa, MasterCard orders provide the following information:

Card#: _____ Expiration Date: _____ Security Code: ____

Signature: _____

Name (print) _____

Address: _____

_____

_____

Telephone #: _____

Subtotal _____

Shipping & Handling _____
$6.00–one book
$1.50 each additional book

Sales Tax _____
(6.5% IL residents only)

Total Due _____